T0211363

HIV CARE

HIV CARE

A Comprehensive Handbook for Providers

Laurie J. Andrews
Laurie B. Novick
and Associates

SAGE Publications
International Educational and Professional Publisher
Thousand Oaks   London   New Delhi

For information address:

SAGE Publications, Inc.
2455 Teller Road
Thousand Oaks, California 91320

SAGE Publications Ltd.
6 Bonhill Street
London EC2A 4PU
United Kingdom

SAGE Publications India Pvt. Ltd.
32 Market
Greater Kailash I
New Delhi 110 048 India

The authors and the publisher of this volume have taken care that the information and recommendations contained herein are accurate and compatible with the standards of practice generally accepted at the time of publication. Nevertheless, it is difficult to ensure that all the information given is entirely accurate in any specific circumstance. Nor can they be considered absolute or universal recommendations. For individual applications, recommendations must be considered in light of the client's clinical condition and their physician's expertise. The authors and publisher disclaim any liability, loss, or damage incurred as a consequence, directly or indirectly, of the use and application of any of the contents of this volume.

Library of Congress Cataloging-in-Publication Data

Andrews, Laurie J.
    HIV care : a comprehensive handbook for providers / Laurie J.
Andrews, Laurie B. Novick, and associates.
        p.   cm.
    Includes bibliographical references and index.
    ISBN 0-8039-7083-8 (alk. paper). — ISBN 0-8039-7150-8 (pbk. : alk. paper)
    1. AIDS (Disease)—Patients—Care.   I. Novick, Laurie B.
II. Title.
    RC607.A26A48   1995
    362.1'969792—dc20   94-40645

This book is printed on acid-free paper.

95 96 97 98 99   10 9 8 7 6 5 4 3 2

Production Editor: Yvonne Könneker
Copy Editor: Linda Gray
Ventura Typesetter: Janelle LeMaster

Brief Contents

Detailed Contents

Preface

These guidelines are intended as a tool to assist practitioners in their care of people with HIV infection or at risk for HIV. They provide useful information about administering treatments but are in no way a substitute for the sound medical judgments that clinicians must make in caring for individual patients. The information contained in these guidelines reflects the existing body of knowledge regarding HIV care at the time of publication. As new studies continually provide additional information and new treatments continue to be approved, the standard of practice may change. Providers of HIV care must take it upon themselves to stay current on these changing developments in care.

HIV Guidelines
Philosophy Statement

These guidelines are a resource to assist primary care providers in giving comprehensive, up-to-date and supportive care to people with HIV disease. They are written within the context of a rapidly evolving knowledge base on HIV and its management.

The spectrum of illness that HIV presents begins at the moment of infection. The philosophy of viewing HIV as a chronic, manageable disease is woven throughout this manual. Data strongly support early intervention in concert with aggressive diagnosis and management. Working in partnership with patients to involve them in decision making regarding their care has been shown to positively affect patient survival. These elements form the cornerstone of quality HIV care.

Although HIV is a life-threatening condition, it is important to do everything possible to enhance the patient's quality of life. This means viewing the patient as someone *living* with HIV and taking seriously *all* medical problems that matter to the patient. Life management issues such as safe housing, emotional well-being, and financial stability also have an impact on a person's overall health.

We recognize that HIV disease is not confined solely to the physical being; our experience confirms that it pervades all aspects of a person's life, including the patient's entire support system. With such a balance in mind, we have adopted a holistic approach and have strived to address all aspects of life. We encourage all providers to integrate this philosophy as they work with people with HIV.

A common thread woven throughout this guideline is the belief that a collaborative approach results in the best care. Individuals from a wide variety of disciplines contributed to this document to make it as comprehensive in focus as possible.

A Special Thank-You

We would like to offer our deepest thanks to our chief medical consultants, Larry B. Broisman, MD, Director of the HIV/AIDS Clinic and Associate Attending, Section of General Internal Medicine, at Hartford Hospital, and John D. Shanley, MD, Director of the Division of Infectious Diseases at the University of Connecticut Health Center. We are deeply indebted to Dr. Broisman for his extraordinary availability to answer our every question and for the countless hours he spent contributing to the medical section and reviewing each draft of this book. We also extend our appreciation to Dr. Shanley for marshaling the medical expertise of the Greater Hartford medical community and making it available to us. This book would not have been possible without their support.

Acknowledgments

These HIV Health Care Guidelines are the result of a regionwide volunteer effort of more than 50 individuals, including physicians, nurses, social workers, AIDS service providers, and others in the community. We extend a heartfelt thank-you to all who have donated so generously of their time and energy to bring this project to fruition.

We wish to acknowledge the many individuals and organizations who contributed to the health care guidelines.

Our chief medical editors: Larry B. Broisman, MD, and John D. Shanley, MD.

Our many writers: Clara Acosta-Glynn, MSW, Social Worker/HIV Counselor, University of Connecticut Pediatric HIV Program; Laurie Andrews, RN, AIDS Coordinator, Hartford Hospital; Maritza Angulo, Coordinator of Support Services, Project Mercy; Marie Hebert Begley, RN, Mount Sinai Hospital/University of Connecticut Burgdorf Clinic; Virginia Berrien, RNC, MSN, Clinical Coordinator, University of Connecticut Pediatric HIV Program; Larry Broisman, MD, Chairman, HIV/AIDS Committee, Director, AIDS Clinic, Hartford Hospital; Jane Burgess, RN, MS, AIDS Consultant, Connecticut State Department of Education; Winston A. Campbell, MD, Associate Professor, Maternal-Fetal Medicine, University of Connecticut Health Center; Susan Cavilliere, RN, BA, CIC, Infection Control Practitioner, Manchester Memorial Hospital; Kathy Clarke, BA, MS, AIDS Coordinator, Disability Determination

xxi

Services; Freddie Close, RN, HIV Coordinator, Visiting Nurse Community Care, Inc.; Kieran A. Cooper, MD, Community Health Services; Helen Crowe, MD, Assistant Director, Infectious Disease, Hartford Hospital; Debbie Dean, MSW, CISW, Pediatric Social Worker, Mount Sinai Outpatient Services; Victor D'Lugin, PhD, Board Member, Hartford Gay and Lesbian Health Collective; Judy Ebetts, MS, APRN, CS, Psychiatric Clinical Nurse Specialist, Hartford Hospital; Lola Elliott-Hugh, MS, BS, Director, AIDS Legal Network for Connecticut; Lisa Fenton, MS, Substance Abuse Counselor, Hartford Hospital; Susan Garten, JD, Legal Aid Society of Hartford; Michael Gerber, MD, Professor, Director, Pediatric Infectious Disease, University of Connecticut Health Center; Brian R. Goodrich, MSW, HIV/AIDS Coordinator, Mount Sinai Hospital/University of Connecticut Outpatient Clinic; Bruce Gould, MD, Medical Director/Chief, Community Medicine, Mount Sinai Hospital/University of Connecticut Health Center Outpatient Services, Chairman, Ambulatory Services, Saint Francis Hospital and Medical Center, Professor of Medicine, University of Connecticut; Manfred Henry, Former Director, Chemical Dependency Program, Community Health Services; Valerie Holcomb, APRN, Pediatric Clinic, Hartford Hospital; Ned Jaroszewski, MD, Director, Emergency Psychiatry Service, Hartford Hospital; George Johnson, MD, Former Director, Pediatric HIV Program, Professor, University of Connecticut Health Center; Patricia Joyce, MD, Medical Director, Pediatric Clinic, Mount Sinai Hospital/Burgdorf Clinic; Jerilynn Lamb-Pagone, MSN, RN, CS, Assistant Chief of Mental Health Nursing Services, Connecticut Department of Mental Health; Shawn Lang, Membership Services Coordinator, Connecticut AIDS Residence Coalition; Sharon Lappen, BS, Eligibility Services, Manchester Department of Income Maintenance; Michael Levinson, Division Chief, Acute Services Division, Capitol Region Mental Health; Richard Melchreit, MD, Medical Associate, AIDS Section, Connecticut Department of Health Services; John Merz, M.Div., Executive Director, AIDS Ministries Program of Connecticut; Ellen Nestler, MD, Assistant Professor of Medicine, Site Director, UCPCIM Residency, Mount Sinai Hospital/Burgdorf Clinic; Laurie Novick, MHSA, BSW, Coordinator, Greater Hartford HIV Action Initiative; Graciella Quinones, MSW, Mental Health Clinician, Community Health Center of Meriden; Christine Ratzel, MSW, Staff Social Worker, Rockville General Hospital; Phillip Richmond, MS, CADC, Assistant Director, Hartford Dispensary; James Robinson, MD, Associate Professor, Pediatrics, University of Connecticut Health Center; Jack Ross, MD, Director, Hartford Hospital AIDS Program; Eyton Rubinstein, MD, Infectious Disease, Saint Francis Hospital and Medical

Center; Gary E. Savill, PhD, Director of Psychology, Capitol Region Mental Health Center; John Shanley, MD, Director, Division of Infectious Disease, Professor of Medicine, University of Connecticut Health Center; Robert Siegel, MD, Medical Oncologist, Hartford Hospital; Margaret Spencer, APRN, Nurse Practitioner, HIV Clinic, Hartford Hospital; Lillian Tamayo, ACSW, Executive Director, Capitol Region Mental Health Center; Kathy Tummillo, RNCS, BSN, Nursing Health Care Consultant, Manchester Area Network on AIDS/Manchester Health Department/Greater Hartford AIDS Collaborative; Lorraine Wells, MA, RNC, Clinical Research Facilitator, University of Connecticut Pediatric HIV Program; Charles Wilber, M.Ed., Coordinator, Substance Abuse Services, Hartford Hospital; Rick Wilkinson, RN, MS, Coordinator, Addiction Services, Mount Sinai Hospital; Pam Williams, RN, Visiting Nurse Association Hospice, Hartford Branch; Barbara Zebrowski, MA, Case Work Supervisor, Project Start.

We extend grateful appreciation to those who reviewed and edited early versions of this document: Larry Broisman, MD, Helen Crowe, MD, Mary Dewald, Joseph J. Klimek, MD, Richard Melchreit, MD, John Merz, M.Div., Paul Pickard, Jack Ross, MD, John Shanley, MD, Margaret Spencer, NP, Kathy Tummillo, NP.

A special thank you to Nancy Post, Sara Ellison, Alice M. Kelly, Pat Baxa, and Deborah Forestiere of Northeast Utilities and to Mary Dewald, Judy Keane, Keisha Holloway, Barbara Sullivan, Carol Ross, and Shawn Lang.

We are grateful to the Hartford County Medical Association, particularly Richard Melchreit, MD, the Capitol Area Health Consortium, John Meehan of Hartford Hospital, and Les Cutler of the University of Connecticut Medical School for their support of this project.

We would like to acknowledge the Greater Hartford HIV Action Initiative, particularly Initiative Steering Committee Chairman William B. Ellis, Chairman of Northeast Utilities, for making this project possible. The unique partnership of corporations, health care institutions, grassroots organizations, and people living with HIV who comprise the Greater Hartford HIV Action Initiative has made this book possible.

List of Acronyms
and Abbreviations

ABGs	arterial blood gases
ACTG	AIDS Clinical Trials Group
ADA	The Americans With Disabilities Act of 1990
ADC	AIDS dementia complex
ADLs	activities of daily living
AFB	acid-fast bacilli
AFDC	Aid to Families With Dependent Children
ANC	absolute neutrophil count
ARC	AIDS-related complex
BAL	bronchoalveolar lavage
BCG	bacile Calmette-Guerin (tuberculosis vaccine)
BDI	Beck Depression Inventory
β-HCG	beta-human chorionic gonadotropin
bid	twice a day
BUN	blood urea nitrogen
CAT	computerized axial tomography
CBC	complete blood count
CD	communicable disease

CDC	Centers for Disease Control
CD4	helper cells
CIN	cervical intraepithelial neoplasia
CMV	cytomegalovirus
CNS	central nervous system
COBRA	Consolidated Omnibus Budget Reconciliation Act
CPK	creatinine phosphokinase
C&S	culture and sensitivity
CSF	cerebrospinal fluid
CVS	cardiovascular system
CXR	chest X-ray
DNR	do not resuscitate
DOT	direct observed therapy
DPT	diptheria, pertussis, and tetanus
DRS	Dementia Rating Scale
DSPN	distal symmetric polyneuropathy
DTH	delayed-type hypersensitivity
d.t.'s	delirium tremens
ELISA	enzyme-linked immunosorbent assay
ERCP	endoscopic retrograde cholangiopancreatiography
ERISA	The Employee Retirement Income Security Act
ESR	erythrocyte sedimentation rate
FDA	Food and Drug Administration
FTA-ABS	fluorescent treponemal antibody-absorption test
G-CSF or GM-CSF	granulocyte stimulating factors
GI	gastrointestinal
G6PD	glucose-6-phosphate dehydrogenase
gtts	drops
HBcAb	hepatitis B core antibody
HBsAg	hepatitis B surface antigen
HBV	hepatitis B virus
HIB	*Hemophilus influenzae* Type B
HiBCV	*Hemophilus influenzae* Type B conjugate vaccine
HPV	human papillomavirus
IDU	injection drug user
Ig	immunoglobulin
IgG	immunoglobulin G
IM	intramuscular

IND	investigational new drugs
INH	Isoniazid
IPV	inactivated polio vaccine
ITP	idiopathic thrombocytopenia purpura
IU	international units
IUGR	intrauterine growth retardation
IV	intravenous
IVIG	intravenous immune globulin
KS	Kaposi's sarcoma
LFTs	liver function tests
LDH	lactate dehydrogenase
LIP	lymphocytic interstitial pneumonia
LP	lumbar puncture
MAC	*Mycobacterium avium* complex
MDRTB	multidrug resistant tuberculosis
MMR	measles, mumps, rubella
MRI	magnetic resonance imaging
MSAFP	maternal serum alpha-fetoprotein
NHL	non-Hodgkin's lymphoma
NIH	National Institutes of Health
NSAIDs	nonsteroidal anti-inflammatory drugs
O&P	ova and parasites
OPV	oral polio vaccine
PCP	*Pneumocystis carinii* pneumonia
PGL	persistent generalized lymphadenopathy
PID	pelvic inflammatory disease
PML	progressive multifocal leukoencephalopathy
PMNs	polymorphonuclear granulocytes
po	by mouth
PO_2	partial pressure of oxygen
PPD	purified protein derivative (tuberculin skin test)
PUBS	percutaneous umbilical blood sampling
PUVA	psoralen ultraviolet A light
qid	four times a day
RAU	recurrent aphthous ulcers
RBB	transbronchial biopsy
ROS	review of systems
RPR	rapid plasma reagin

RSV	respiratory syncytial virus
Rx	prescription, treatment
SDMT	The Symbol Digit Modalities Test
SLE	systemic lupus erythematosus
SMX	sulfamethoxazole
SNST	Stroop Neuropsychological Screening Test
SOB	short of breath
SSA	Social Security Administration
SSDI	Social Security Disability Insurance
SSI	Supplemental Security Income
STD	sexually transmitted disease
TB	tuberculosis
Td	tetanus-diphtheria
tid	three times a day
TMP	trimethoprim
TNF	tumor necrosis factor
U/A	urinalysis
USP	United States Pharmacopeia
VDRL	Venereal Disease Research Laboratory
VZIG	varicella-zoster immune globulin
VZV	varicella-zoster virus
WBC	white blood cell
ZDV	zidovudine
ZIG	zoster immunoglobulin

List of Brand Names

The following brand names used in the text are registered trademarks. The appearance of any name without designation as proprietary is not to be regarded as a representation by the publisher that it is not a trademark or is not the subject of proprietary rights.

Aristocort®	Heptavax®	Neutrexan®	Septra DS®
Atabrine®	Hivid®	Nizoral®	Sporonox®
Bactrim®	Imodium®	Norpramin®	Trental®
Bactrim DS®	INH®	Pamelor®	Trilafon®
Benadryl®	Kaopectate®	Peridex®	Trimpex®
Cipro®	Kenalog®	Phenergan®	Vancocin®
Compazine®	K-Y Jelly®	Pneumovax®	Vaseline®
Crisco®	Lidex®	Proloprim®	Xylocaine®
Dapsone®	Lomotil®	Pyrazinamide®	Yodoxin®
Daraprim®	Marinol®	Recombivax®	Zerit®
Decadron®	Megace®	Reglan®	Zetar®
Deltasone®	Mepron®	Retrovir®	Shampoo
Diflucan®	Myambutol®	Rifadin®	Zofran®
Elavil®	Mycelex®	Ritalin®	Zovirax®
Flagyl®	Mycobutin®	Selsun Blue®	
Haldol®	Mycostatin®	Septra®	

1

HIV Counseling and Testing

All adult and adolescent patients should be considered potentially at risk of HIV infection. Regardless of marital status, class, race, residence, age, or assumed sexual orientation, assumptions cannot be made about risk for HIV. Providers have the responsibility of raising this issue routinely with patients. Your patient should be interviewed alone and given assurance that everything discussed will be held in strict confidence. Your comfort in discussing these issues in a nonjudgmental manner will facilitate the patient's ability to respond honestly and completely.

Many states have confidentiality laws that outline how information about HIV status must be handled. You can obtain a copy of your state law by contacting your state department of public health.

Testing is often the first step an individual takes in acknowledging his or her risk for HIV. Comprehensive counseling is essential to this process.

Risk Assessment Tool: Making the Decision to Test

Asking your patients the following questions will assist you in determining whether or not HIV antibody testing is indicated:

1. Have you been sexually active within the past 14 years? (If no, go to Question 9). With men, women, or both?

2. Do you believe you have been sexually active only within a mutually monogamous relationship with an uninfected partner during this time? (The patient may be unaware of partner's risk activities; explore this further.)

3. Have you had intercourse (anal/vaginal) without a condom during this time?

4. Have you talked with your partner(s) about his or her (their) risk for HIV?

5. Do you understand what safer sexual practices are? (Ask the patient for a description; correct any misinformation he or she may have.)

6. Do you use safer sex practices now? If yes, ask, "How long have you been doing this? Do you use condoms *every* time?"

7. Do you believe your partner(s) may be (at risk of being) HIV infected? To your knowledge, has he or she (they) had other sexual partners, used needles, tested positive, had a previous sexual partner who was infected, or received blood transfusions or blood products?

8. Do you use drugs/alcohol? If yes, ask, "Do you consistently practice safer sex even when using these substances?"

9. Have you used needles within the past 14 years? Did you ever share needles, cookers, or other drug paraphernalia?

10. Are you using injection drugs now? If yes, ask, "Are you interested in treatment?"

11. Have you received a transfusion of blood or blood products? If so, when and where?

The more risk behaviors that patients engage in, the greater the risk they are of being infected. However, any risk behavior is cause for concern.

Issues Concerning Counseling and Testing

Since the onset of this epidemic, we have learned a great deal about HIV disease. Because HIV can affect anyone, providers should address risk factors and perceptions about personal risk with every patient. Although HIV infection among gay and bisexual men and injection drug users (IDUs) is well documented, infection in women and adolescents has also increased substantially. Women are often unaware of their partners' sexual or drug-using behaviors, which place these women at great risk. Women for whom domestic violence is an issue may be especially unable to confront their partners about risk behaviors or negotiate safer sex practices.

HIV testing raises many complex issues. HIV counseling should offer up-to-date information and an opportunity to explore concerns in a sensitive manner. These two elements are essential to the testing process and *must* be done in person. They are an important first step in assisting those who have HIV to deal with their disease.

Receiving a positive antibody test is the beginning of a journey of learning to live with HIV, one that may be filled with discrimination in employment, housing, insurance coverage, and medical care. In addition, people with HIV may also have to deal with our culture's taboos concerning sexual identity, drug use, sexual behaviors, and death. All of these contribute to the stigma that may be placed on people with HIV.

Understanding these issues, as well as being sensitive to cultural and linguistic differences are key in developing trusting and successful relationships with patients.

If a patient's primary language is not English, even if he or she understands a little English, the provider should offer information and allow for questions in the patient's primary language, using a translator when appropriate.

Culture, ethnicity, religion, class, sexual orientation, and gender affect a patient's reaction to his or her illness. This includes reactions to pain, views of male and female roles, the importance and inclusion of family, the absence of peer support, and reluctance to access available support. These factors can also contribute to a man's reluctance to use condoms or a couple's reluctance about contraception in general.

Differences are also manifested when discussing or describing sexual behaviors. For example, *oral sex* is not a term used by all people. It is helpful to ask people how they describe sexual behaviors. Some women may also have difficulty discussing sexual matters with any male, including the health care provider.

The responsibilities that women carry as the primary caregivers in their families often affect their ability to come to terms with their illness. Concerns about bearing children as well as caring for children they already have are issues that need to be addressed.

Knowing how a patient became infected may help providers understand issues that the patient may be facing. However, it may take time and the development of a trusting relationship for the patient to share this information with his or her provider. Finally, it is important for you, as a provider, to identify your own biases so that you can approach the patient with a nonjudgmental attitude. Only then will the door open to working with the patient on his or her health and well-being.

Pretest Counseling

Counseling in language that is direct, simple, and familiar to patients is critical. The following is written in language recommended for use when counseling patients.

DEFINE HIV/AIDS

AIDS is a disease caused by a virus (HIV) that damages the immune system. Our bodies try to fight that infection by making antibodies that can be found in the blood. HIV antibodies are a sign that the virus has entered the bloodstream. People can live with HIV, symptom free, for long periods of time, or they may become sicker in time and develop life-threatening illnesses.

EXPLAIN THE IMMUNE SYSTEM

The immune system is the part of your body that protects you from infection. The immune system is made up of white blood cells and antibodies, whose job is to fight infection. HIV attacks a kind of white blood cell called a *T-cell*—a very important cell in the immune system.

IDENTIFY RISK ACTIVITIES

Risk activities include having unprotected sex or sharing needles or *any* paraphernalia that may contain blood, such as cocaine straws and cookers. Judgment and self-control are likely to be altered while under the influence of any drug, including alcohol.

TRANSMISSION AND PREVENTION

See "Transmission and Risk-Reducing Practices" later in this chapter.

WHAT A NEGATIVE TEST MEANS

Antibodies to the virus are not present in your blood at this time. There are two possible reasons for this:

- You have not been infected with the virus.

TABLE 1.1 Spectrum of HIV Illness

HIV Infection, No Symptoms	Symptomatic HIV Disease	AIDS
	Fevers	Opportunistic infection
	Night sweats	Cancers
	Weight loss	Wasting
	Loss of appetite	AIDS dementia complex
	Diarrhea	Recurrent pneumonia
	Rashes	Cervical cancer
	Thrush	Tuberculosis
	Fatigue	T-cells > 200
	Skin changes	
	Infections	
	Swollen glands	
400 to 1,000 T-cells	400 to 200 T-cells	400 to 0 T-cells
Little or no damage to immune system or other parts of the body	Some symptoms due to at least some damage to immune system	Severe symptoms from serious damage to immune system and other parts of the body

- You have been infected with the virus but have not yet produced antibodies. (There is a window period of 6 to 12 weeks since the last risk behavior, but it may be as long as 1 year or more in rare cases.)

WHAT A POSITIVE TEST MEANS

- Antibodies to the virus are found in your blood.
- You have been infected with HIV and can pass it on to other people through vaginal, anal, and, possibly, oral sex or by sharing needles.
- If you are pregnant, you can pass the virus to your baby during pregnancy, birth, and after birth through breast-feeding.
- You have HIV disease but may not have symptoms at this time.
- It is possible, but *very* unlikely, that the test result is a false-positive.

HOW THE TEST CAN HELP

- If the test is negative, you can learn ways to better protect yourself and your partner(s) from getting the virus in the future.
- If the test is positive, you can work with your doctor to better take care of yourself. (Table 1.1 shows the spectrum of HIV illness.)

- You can learn how not to pass the virus on to others.
- You can use the information to help make decisions about medical care, pregnancy, drug treatment, and other issues.
- If you are pregnant, you can get more counseling, arrange for special prenatal care, consider starting antiretroviral therapy, and make other medical arrangements.

CONFIDENTIALITY/DISCRIMINATION

- You do not have to take the test. If you are concerned about confidentiality and/or insurance, options for testing are available at sites that provide free and anonymous (names are not used) or confidential testing.
- If you have the test done in an office or a clinic, results are private, but they can be shared with health providers, insurance companies or Medicaid to pay for services, and other health care institutions where you receive care.
- Potential exists for (a) discrimination based on HIV status in housing and employment; (b) loss or estrangement from family, friends, and/or coworkers; or (c) problems with insurance companies.

ASSESSING COPING SKILLS

- How will you feel and what will you do if the test result is negative? (Reinforce the need to begin or continue safer sex practices.)
- How will you feel and what will you do if the result is positive? In what ways have you dealt with stress in the past? Who is available to support you?

NOTE: If the patient tests positive, help him or her decide how to inform sexual or needle-sharing partners. Assistance may be available through your state or local health department.

Posttesting Counseling

NOTE: Test results must never be given by telephone!

WHEN THE TEST RESULT IS NEGATIVE

- Review what a negative test means (see "Pretest Counseling").
- Review transmission and risk reduction practices, including safer needle and sexual practices (see "Transmission and Risk-Reducing Practices").

WHEN THE TEST RESULT IS POSITIVE

> *NOTE:* When giving a positive test result, be sure to evaluate suicide potential or the need for crisis intervention.

Typically, learning of HIV seropositivity raises immediate feelings of being overwhelmed and isolated. Posttest counseling is an essential piece of the process of helping patients learn to live with HIV infection. Hope should be fostered and information presented in a way that encourages living with HIV. Having information empowers those infected to make decisions about their health and allows them to maintain some control over their lives. It is also helpful to those who are newly diagnosed and feeling overwhelmed to be encouraged to follow a philosophy of "taking it one day at a time" so that coping with this devastating information feels more manageable.

Explore how the patient may be feeling. Patients commonly react by expressing a range of feelings, such as guilt, regret, relief, and fear of death, and by asking, "Why me?" HIV illness can present an opportunity to deal with unresolved issues, which can have a negative effect on quality of life. *Your* attitude is important in shaping patients' responses to their test results. Stressing the following is helpful:

- This is not a death sentence.
- We can work together as a team.
- A positive attitude can have a positive impact on the course of this disease.
- There are reasons to be hopeful; new drugs for treating and managing HIV illness are in constant development.
- This is a disease, not a punishment.

REVIEW WHAT A POSITIVE TEST MEANS
(see "Pretest Counseling")

- Antibodies to the virus are found in your blood.
- You have been infected with HIV and can pass it on to other people through vaginal, anal, and possibly oral sex or by sharing needles.
- You can pass the virus to your baby during pregnancy, birth, and through breast-feeding.
- Whether or not you have symptoms, you have HIV disease.

Posttest Counseling Checklist

The following points should be covered with patients in the posttest counseling sessions:

_____ Your immune system protects you from infection through white blood cells and antibodies.

_____ HIV infection/AIDS is caused by a virus.

_____ The virus that causes AIDS damages the immune system and other cells in your body.

_____ If you are HIV infected, you usually make antibodies to fight this infection within 6 to 12 weeks, but sometimes it may take longer. It is the antibodies that we look for in your blood when we test for HIV.

_____ HIV antibodies are a sign that the virus is living in your body and that you can give it to other people through blood, semen, and vaginal fluid.

_____ One of the cells most damaged by the AIDS virus is called the *T-cell.* It is a kind of white blood cell. T-cells play an important role in your immune system.

_____ HIV is a chronic, manageable disease, and there are different stages of the disease. Generally, the more damaged your immune system is, the more likely you are to develop symptoms and infections. It is possible to have a very damaged immune system and to have few or no symptoms. However, regardless of your symptoms, you are still susceptible to infections.

_____ When you are first infected, you may have few or no symptoms because you have little or no damage to your immune system.

_____ As the virus stays in the body longer, it tends to damage the immune system. This damage can lead to development of symptoms.

_____ As the virus stays in the body even longer, it may do serious damage to your immune system and other parts of your body, making you susceptible to serious problems.

_____ Whether or not you have symptoms, you are considered infected and infectious (able to give the virus to others) for life.

_____ Normally, your T-cell level is between 600 and 1,000. As the virus damages your immune system, your T-cell level begins to drop. Usually people don't develop symptoms until their T-cell level falls below 400.

_____ Taking care of yourself can affect the course of your disease:

Good nutrition	Stay away from people with colds and flu.
Sleep	Cook meat and eggs well.
Exercise	Wear gloves when changing cat litter or bird cages.
Decrease stress	Alcohol and other drugs can damage your immune system.

_____ Infection control

- Don't share your toothbrush and/or razor—they may have blood on them.
- It is OK to wash laundry and dishes with others'.
- Use bleach to clean blood spills on surfaces (diluted to a 1:10 strength, 1 part bleach to 9 parts water).
- Inform sexual and needle-sharing partners about your HIV status (you can get assistance in doing this).
- Do not donate blood, sperm, organs, or other body tissues.
- HIV may be transmitted in pregnancy, at birth, or through breast milk.

_____ Diagnostic testing

- It is important to know the level of damage the virus may have done to your immune system. Until further diagnostic tests are done, it is not possible to know how much damage the virus has done. You should also be screened for infections for which you are at risk. Tests are done to look for immune system damage and the presence of other infections such as sexually transmitted diseases and tuberculosis.

_____ Treatment options

- Based on your level of disease and your underlying health, you may be offered antiviral medication or medication to prevent infections. You should also have a yearly flu vaccine and a pneumococcal vaccine every 6 years.

_____ Identifying support

- It may be helpful to plan who you will share information about your HIV status with and how you will share it.
- Services such as support groups, buddies, and help applying for financial assistance, housing, and legal programs and so on may be available through community-based AIDS service organizations.

Transmission and Risk-Reducing Practices

NOTE: Individuals should be supported in their right to choose not to have sex with others or to practice safer sex.

SAFER SEX

- Safer sexual practices involve sexual partners keeping their blood, semen, pre-ejaculate, and vaginal secretions from entering each other's bodies.

- Differing sexual behaviors carry different levels of risk, depending on how likely they are to allow blood, semen, pre-ejaculate, and vaginal secretions to enter a partner's body.
- Understanding levels of risk is important for making informed choices about how much risk is acceptable.
- The most important way of reducing risk of transmission is wearing latex condoms for anal and/or vaginal sex.
- Individuals should use a water-based lubricant, such as K-Y Jelly, and never one that is oil based, such as hand lotion, Vaseline, or Crisco.
- Condoms should never be stored in a glove compartment or back pocket because they can dry out.
- Space should be left at the tip of the condom to contain semen. Air should be squeezed out of the tip.
- The condom should be removed immediately after ejaculation.
- Using condoms with spermicide, such as nonoxynol-9, may offer additional protection; nonoxynol-9 appears to have viricidal activity. However, because nonoxynol-9 causes irritation in some people, it is possible that it may actually increase the risk of infection for those individuals. Nonoxynol-9 should be applied to the wrist before using to check for irritation; if irritation occurs, it should definitely not be used.
- Most sexual practices are considered less risky than unprotected anal or vaginal intercourse. All forms of oral sex and sexual activity in which there is a possibility of blood or semen entering the body through broken skin may pose some risk. Using latex barriers (condoms, gloves, finger cots) will further reduce this risk.
- Even if both partners are infected, they should practice safer sex so as not to reinfect each other.
- A truly mutually monogamous relationship between uninfected partners carries no risk of infection. However, there are two problems with relying on monogamy. First, monogamy is not always assured. Second, one partner may already be infected.

LEVELS OF SAFER SEX

- Absolutely safe (OK)
  — Kissing, masturbation, humping, oral sex on a man with a condom, oral sex on a woman with a dental dam or plastic wrap, rimming (oral-anal) with a dental dam or plastic wrap, finger sex with latex gloves or finger cots on, external water sports (urinating on someone), touching, massage, fantasy
- Reasonably safe (OK)
  — Vaginal intercourse with a condom, anal intercourse with a condom

- May be risky (think about)
  — Oral sex on a man without a condom, masturbation on open sores and/or broken skin, oral sex on a woman without a barrier, rimming without a barrier
- High risk (don't do)
  — Vaginal intercourse without a condom, anal intercourse without a condom, oral sex without a barrier on a woman while she has her period, internal water sports (urinating into a body cavity), fisting without gloves and a lubricant
- Causes of impaired judgment
  — Drugs (amphetamines, heroin, amyl nitrite [poppers], cocaine, pot, and so on)
  — Alcohol

SHARING NEEDLES AND PARAPHERNALIA

- Works should be cleaned (needles, syringes, cookers) by flushing needles and syringes twice with bleach and rinsing twice with water; sharing of needles and cookers or straws when shooting or snorting drugs should be avoided.
- Needles purchased on the street should never be considered clean, even if packaged.

OTHER RISK-REDUCTION PRACTICES

- Razors and toothbrushes should not be shared.
- If infected, blood, organs, sperm, or other body tissues should not be donated.
- A bleach solution to clean blood and other body fluid spills should be used (diluted to a 1:10 strength, 1 part bleach to 9 parts water).
- Review risk of transmitting HIV in pregnancy, at birth, or by breast-feeding.

HIV Counseling and Test Sites

Your state department of health can provide you with a list of anonymous and confidential sites for HIV testing.

2

Working With Chemically
Dependent Patients

When treating addicts who are HIV infected, it is important to remember that addiction is their primary illness; often, it is more immediately life threatening than HIV. This section is intended as a guide in working with the patient who is chemically dependent. The potential medical problems associated with alcohol and drug use are numerous and complex. Patients using alcohol and other drugs may have the same diseases as those who are not users. The natural history of coincidental illness is, however, frequently affected by their use of alcohol and drugs and by their lifestyles. Certain medical problems are found to be direct or indirect complications from alcohol and drug use in the HIV-infected patient, such as seizures, endocarditis, or malnutrition.

Caring for the active addict can be very frustrating. The impulse to lecture, punish, frighten, or control these patients is natural but usually counterproductive. Friends and family members may have already exhausted all these approaches in an attempt to effect some change. Although you have no control over the patient's behavior, your consistent encouragement to take active steps to deal with the addiction may eventually prove successful. Interactions producing the best outcomes are direct and open, educating patients about their medical problems in a nonjudgmental manner. Conceptualizing and communicating about addictive disorders as a disease in a medical model, rather than a problem in the moral domain, will allow you to gain some distance from personal feelings. This will enable these patients to interact with you as a provider, not as a parent figure.

Finally, alcoholism and drug dependence are not hopeless illnesses. Chemically dependent persons can and do recover. An appropriate referral to a detox, methadone, or recovery program can turn someone's life around if he or she is ready to make a change. HIV diagnosis is often the crisis needed to catalyze a change in drug-using behavior. Treatment is always recommended. If you need assistance in working with these patients, contact the substance abuse representative of your institution or call a local drug treatment agency.

Tips for Understanding
the Addict With HIV Disease

- Addicts who are HIV infected may use the crisis of diagnosis to confront their addiction realistically for the very first time. It is important to take an active approach in encouraging the addict to seek drug treatment and pursue active medical care for his or her HIV.

- Addiction is an incurable but treatable illness affecting the body, mind, and spirit. It is chronic, progressive, and life threatening.

- Feelings of shame, inadequacy, anger, depression, and anxiety often accompany addiction. If someone is trying to become clean after a long period of using, it is likely that these suppressed feelings will surface. Once they decide to pursue treatment or enter recovery, patients are likely to feel both emotionally and physically worse before they feel better.

- Typically, addicts operate from a need for instant gratification. They may enter treatment or show up at a medical appointment *if* it is available at the moment they feel that they need it. Often, this tendency to meet the need of the moment contributes to noncompliance and an inability to follow through on agreements despite the best of intentions.

- Addicts often tend to isolate. When they enter recovery, they may need to learn new ways of relating to others and how to live responsibly. Coaching and support are necessary to prevent relapse.

- The risk of relapse is always present. Individuals commonly relapse several times during the recovery process and may be at particular risk when learning of their HIV status. Support and reinforcement of continued recovery efforts are important; condemning a patient for slipping is generally counterproductive. Patients should be encouraged to seek additional support during crisis points of HIV progression—for example, learning of their HIV seropositivity, development of new infections, and so on. Signs that a patient is heading toward relapse include increased isolation and a tendency to blame others for negative feelings or life circumstances. Point out when you think that patients are in danger. Stress the importance of a drug-free lifestyle in maintaining a strong immune system.

- Be open to being surprised. Some of your patients will be completely different people once they are able to get their addiction under control.

Guide to Substance Use History

A thorough drug history is essential for obtaining a complete picture of the patient. This should include *all* drugs, licit and illicit, including alcohol and tobacco.

In discussing each drug, the following should be noted:

- Class of drug
- Age at first use
- Past and current use
- Mode of administration (injection, oral, inhalation)
- Frequency of use and estimated dose
- Development of tolerance (need to increase the dose to achieve the same effect)
- Presence or absence of withdrawal symptoms on discontinuation
- Source (street, prescription, multiple prescriptions, etc.)
- Alleged purpose of use (to get high; to relieve pain, anxiety, insomnia, etc.; "What does the stuff do for you?")
- Motivation, if any, to be drug free ("Why are you here?")
- Approximate date of last use

Substance Abuse

Indicators of substance abuse include the following:

- Continued use of the drug despite its having a negative effect on social, occupational, psychological, or physical aspects of life
- Recurrent use of the drug in situations when use is physically hazardous (e.g., driving while intoxicated)

- Persistence of symptoms for at least 1 month or symptoms occurring repeatedly over a longer period of time

Substance abuse is distinguished from addiction by the lack of physiological signs of withdrawal when the drug is unavailable.

Alcohol Abuse

EARLY IDENTIFICATION OF ALCOHOL-RELATED PROBLEMS

Alcohol use occurs on a continuum from social drinking, through the gradual development of a drinking problem, and finally to the later development of severe medical disorders. Early identification may prove difficult. One must look at a wide range of indications, including psychosocial, medical, and laboratory findings, from which a composite picture emerges. No single finding is diagnostic. As the number of indications suggestive of alcohol-related problems increases, the more likely it is that problematic alcohol use will be identified. Late identification is fairly simple because heavy alcohol consumption is linked with disease entities such as liver disease, peripheral neuropathy, and Wernicke-Korsakoff's syndrome.

EARLY INDICATORS

- Heavy drinking, more than six drinks per day (780g/day ethanol)
- Self-expressed concern about drinking
- Concern expressed by family and/or friends about patient's drinking
- Intellectual impairment
- Eating lightly or skipping meals when drinking
- Drinking quickly; increased tolerance
- Accidents in which drinking is involved
- Tardiness or absence from work because of drinking
- Social life revolves around drinking
- Attempts to cut down on drinking have had limited success
- Frequent use of alcohol to deal with stress, anxiety, depression
- Frequent drinking during the workday (for example, at lunch break)
- Heavy smoking

SIGNS AND SYMPTOMS

- Trauma (e.g., multiple healed rib fractures on X-ray)
- Surgical scars
- Hand tremor
- Smells of alcohol during the day
- Dyspepsia
- Morning nausea and vomiting
- Recurrent diarrhea
- Pancreatitis
- Hepatomegaly
- Elevated liver enzymes and other laboratory abnormalities
- Polyuria
- Impotence
- Palpitations
- Hypertension
- Insomnia, nightmares

A simple screening tool, such as the CAGE (shown next), when used routinely is diagnostically accurate. Physicians can question the patient to elicit the following:

C	Patient feels the need to cut down on drinking.
A	Patient is annoyed by criticism of his or her drinking.
G	Patient feels guilty about drinking.
E	Patient drinks first thing in morning (eye opener).

Even one of these responses calls for further investigation; two increase the probability of problematic alcohol use substantially.

Chemical Dependence

Chemical dependence requires that some symptoms have persisted for at least 1 month or have occurred repeatedly over a longer period of time. Diagnosis is made when the patient exhibits at least three of the following:

- Uses the substance in large amounts or over a longer period than originally intended
- Recognizes that the substance use is excessive and has attempted to reduce or control it but has been unable to do so

- Spends a great deal of time in activities necessary to procure the substance, taking it, or recovering from its effects
- Is unable to effectively fulfill role obligations (e.g., employment, parenting, etc.) due to either intoxication or withdrawal symptoms
- Gives up important social, occupational, or recreational activities because of substance use
- Develops tolerance (needs increasing amounts of the substance to achieve the same effect)
- Develops withdrawal symptoms after cessation or reduction of intake of the substance
- Uses the substance to relieve or avoid withdrawal symptoms

Detoxification

If a patient is ready for help, it may be appropriate to refer him or her to a detox or drug and/or alcohol treatment program. It may be dangerous for patients to attempt detoxification on their own, depending on the substances they are using. Detoxification may occur in inpatient settings, outpatient acupuncture clinics, or outpatient methadone clinics. Waiting lists are common. However, depending on the patient's level of disease, it may be possible for you to expedite admission.

Opiate Detoxification

The most common type of opiate dependency is heroin addiction. Discontinuation of daily use will lead to withdrawal symptoms. Withdrawal symptoms usually include sweating, chills, goose bumps, fever, hypertension, nausea, anorexia, and insomnia. Withdrawal from heroin, although extremely uncomfortable, does not pose a medical risk if untreated. With the exceptions of pregnant women and patients with cardiac conditions, most people can safely withdraw cold turkey. A pregnant woman who wants to stop using heroin must get on methadone maintenance until the baby is born. Opiate withdrawal will endanger the fetus in utero. Pregnant women are often given emergency admission to methadone programs.

If a patient is an intermittent user or has not used for 3 or more consecutive days, methadone or clonidine detoxification is generally unnecessary.

Alcohol Detoxification

Discontinuation of daily alcohol use without pharmaceutical intervention may lead to a medical emergency. Alcohol withdrawal is usually medicated prophylactically with Ativan or Librium at an inpatient detox unit. All patients at risk for alcohol withdrawal should be sent to a city or state detox center or, if insured, to a private detox center. Providing Librium at medical outpatient clinics may allow the alcohol abuse to continue. A referral to an inpatient unit will address the problem directly and appropriately.

Cocaine Detoxification

Discontinuation of daily cocaine use, although difficult, does not constitute a medical emergency. Often, patients hospitalized for cocaine dependence are not medicated at all. Acupuncture detoxification is sometimes helpful for patients discontinuing cocaine use.

Tips for Working With
Chemically Dependent Patients

- Withdrawal from drugs and alcohol is best managed in inpatient settings or on an outpatient basis in a day treatment program.
- Withdrawal from heroin is not a medical emergency unless the patient is pregnant. Pregnant women who are in withdrawal should always be referred to a methadone clinic or a local emergency room. Withdrawal symptoms from opioids are much like a severe case of the 5-day flu that lasts until the opiates are out of the patient's system.
- Withdrawal from alcohol or barbiturates can be a medical emergency, particularly if there is a previous history of delirium tremens (d.t.'s) or with early signs of d.t.'s (i.e., increased temperature, tremor, or reports of changes in sensorium). All patients with this history or who are in withdrawal should be referred to a local emergency room.
- Substance abusers who need analgesics should be medicated appropriately according to their level of pain and discomfort. However, prescriptions should be limited to 1 or 2 weeks' duration so they may be monitored closely.
- Patients with substance abuse histories who abuse prescribed medications or report them lost or stolen should not be issued another prescription unless it is a nonaddictive analgesic (e.g., Motrin), or unless they agree to stick to the current medication regime.

- Prescriptions for medications from the benzodiazepine family of drugs (Xanax, Valium, Librium, etc.) should be monitored carefully and only small prescriptions given.
- Medical patients with a substance abuse history who report symptoms of panic, anxiety, thought disorder, or depression should be referred to a local mental health clinic to ascertain whether these are psychiatric symptoms or signs of withdrawal.
- Stay medically focused when treating substance abusers in outpatient settings— otherwise you may be swept up by their chaotic lifestyle. Remain flexible, open, truthful, and vigilant. Become familiar with and use your local drug and alcohol detox and treatment resources.
- Contracts may be helpful in setting up rules and responsibilities for you and your patient. Contracts are agreements between consenting parties. Familiarize yourself with your own responsibilities as well as the patient's. It is important not to use contracts punitively.
- An objective nonjudgmental discussion of the medical problems associated with the patient's drug or alcohol use will have more influence than an authoritative lecture. Your judgments are more easily discounted than the facts.
- Do not take illicit drug and/or alcohol use by patients personally. Your job is to do what you can to treat the medical problem, not to cure the addiction. Your patient's decision to use or not use drugs is out of your control.

3

Working With
"Noncompliant" Patients

When patients do not comply with provider recommendations, by not taking medications as prescribed or not showing up for scheduled appointments, providers may become frustrated. Often, the provider may interpret this behavior as an indication that the patient is not interested in his or her health or may personalize it. However, many reasons may contribute to this apparent lack of compliance. This section is intended to provide insight into the complex issues that play a role in determining the patient's ability to be an active participant in his or her own health care. With this understanding, the provider will be better able to minimize the factors that negatively influence patient follow-through.

The "Noncompliant" Patient

I. EXAMPLES OF "NONCOMPLIANCE"

    A. Not coming to appointments, not making appointments, or arriving very late

    B. Not filling prescriptions

C. Not taking medications as prescribed

D. Not following through on referrals to other services or providers

II. REASONS FOR "NONCOMPLIANCE"

A. Cultural implications: Cultural or religious beliefs often conflict with recommended treatment. Superstitions regarding approaches or practices exist. Misinterpretations from cultural perspectives (e.g., women who ask their partners to use condoms are viewed as being promiscuous or not caring for their partner; issues of mistrust) also exist.

1. The patient may experience feelings of inferiority, frustration, anger, isolation, and cynicism, as well as a lack of adjustment to HIV status.

2. The provider may lack knowledge of cultural issues that might impede compliance—for example, ethnic religious values, spiritism, traditional therapies versus scientific ones, fatalism, respect, lack of involvement of men (in a culture where men play a big role), family roles and dynamics, nutrition.

B. Personality

1. Personality traits that come between patient needs and ability to comply with treatment (e.g., passive personalities)

2. Personality disorders or mental health problems (e.g., delusional, paranoid disorders, etc.)

3. Behavior traits, such as drug or alcohol use and/or abuse

4. Passive-aggressive behavior as a response to perceived provider lack of understanding

5. Mental retardation, dementia, or illiteracy (not being able to understand prescriptions, doses, or how to obtain them at the pharmacy)

C. Socioeconomics: Poverty, class, and social group issues affect ability to follow through with treatment.

1. Patients may experience feelings of inferiority; live in poverty; lack education; feel powerless to influence changes; be unable to prioritize needs, provide for day-to-day survival, or meet nutritional needs; have no phone or transportation; be homeless; be imprisoned.

2. The provider may be judgmental about poverty, race, class, culture, gender, sexual orientation, addiction, and so on.

D. Difficulties in accessing the health system

1. Long waits at the office or clinic, language barriers, lack of transportation or difficulty in using the existing transportation system, lack of family/community support (no child care, not being able to disclose HIV status)

2. Inability to negotiate the system in the presence of multiple medical, social, and emotional problems

    3. Lack of continuity of providers

  E. Fears: Unstated fears on the part of both the patient and the provider serve as stumbling blocks to a successful patient-provider partnership.

    1. The patient may experience fear of the disease, the provider, or the institution.

    2. The provider may experience fear of HIV infection, patient behaviors (drug use, psychological behavior, sexual identity or practices), and patient's lack of financial means to pay provider or inadequate insurance.

  F. Active substance abuse (see Chapter 2)

III. CONSEQUENCES OF "NONCOMPLIANCE"

  A. Health care is sought only when there is a crisis.

  B. Patient's condition may deteriorate in absence of ongoing health care.

  C. Available resources may burn out due to misuse and/or duplication of services.

  D. Noncompliance may result in increased cost to system.

  E. Noncompliance may contribute to patient and/or provider feelings of frustration and mistrust.

  F. Patient may become defensive due to feelings of powerlessness.

  G. Patient and provider may engage in a power struggle detrimental to the patient-provider relationship.

IV. APPROACHES FOR REDUCING "NONCOMPLIANCE"

  A. Allow the patient to participate in making treatment decisions.

  B. Determine how critical it is for a patient to follow a particular course of treatment when he or she is resistant.

  C. Present all possible treatments, including their side effects or consequences.

  D. Support partial compliance and point out the importance of further compliance.

  E. Assist the patient with developing an understanding of chosen treatment options vis-à-vis other treatment options.

  F. Patients have the right to refuse treatment; this is not necessarily noncompliance.

  G. Recognize the potential for problems before they occur.

    1. Obtain previous medical *and* compliance history.

    2. Identify patient's coping mechanisms (e.g., passive or self-destructive behaviors, fear of accomplishment, need for attention).

  H. Develop a plan of action

    1. Educate the patient about the way the health care system operates and identify noncompliant behavior.

2. Encourage active patient participation in decision making, particularly regarding treatment.
3. Develop a contract. Set limits with clear expectations and defined roles and responsibilities.
4. Be aware that the health care system and providers may intimidate patients.
5. Identify community resources for patient support.

4

Mental Health, Psychosocial, and Spiritual Issues

HIV disease profoundly affects all aspects of one's life. Understanding the psychosocial issues affecting a patient enhances your ability to work effectively together. Patients' emotional responses to HIV play an important role in their ability to follow through on treatment recommendations and actively participate in their own care as well as affect their quality of life.

Patients' attitudes about their disease determine how they live with HIV. A positive attitude appears to be correlated with improved survival. Hope plays an especially important role. A negative attitude, particularly one characterized by hopelessness, fear, and shame, appears to have a negative effect on health, quality of life, and survival.

Your attitude can significantly shape how patients see themselves in relationship to their disease and their ability to maintain hope. Knowing how patients have coped with stressful situations in the past will give you a good idea of how they are likely to cope with HIV. Direct questioning about their coping history will provide you with useful information. Referral for appropriate psychological and emotional support may be in order. However, some patients most in need of this assistance may be least able to accept it. Continued encouragement from you over time to take advantage of available resources may ultimately result in success.

Mental Health Issues

Access to mental health services is critical for people with HIV. Accessing services for people who are dually or triply diagnosed with a psychiatric and/or substance abuse history and HIV presents complex challenges. Those who cannot afford to access private services often have an especially difficult time getting their mental health needs met.

Throughout the course of HIV disease, patients have differing mental health needs. These range from the need for assistance in coping with crises such as diagnosis, hospitalization, physical decline, or rejection by significant others to evaluation and management of dementia, organic psychosis, organic affective disorders, and organic personality disorders.

A broad spectrum of mental health services is needed, including support groups, brief treatment, long-term therapeutic counseling, anticipatory grief counseling, family intervention, crisis intervention, evaluation of psychiatric manifestations, psychotropic medication management, and acute psychiatric hospitalization.

For optimal patient care, mental health providers should be included as part of the treatment team. They can play a critical role in treatment planning and service provision for patients with psychiatric manifestations, particularly those who need assistance with psychiatric management in order to remain in their homes.

Mental Health Services

Most states offer a broad array of publicly funded mental health services running the gamut from inpatient hospitals to outpatient care, day treatment, vocational rehabilitation, and crisis services. However, these programs may be difficult to access and available only to those with histories of severe psychiatric illness. Often, programs are tailored to meet the needs of specific target populations. Your state's Department of Mental Health or a similar division will be able to provide you with information that is specific to your region.

In addition to publicly funded state services, clinics and private practitioners are a source of mental health services. Some practitioners are willing to see people with HIV on a sliding scale. Specially funded programs exist in some communities to meet the mental health needs of people with HIV.

Psychosocial Responses to HIV Disease

Patient responses to HIV disease are variable. Usually, patients will draw on the same coping mechanisms they have used before. Responses are likely to be intense and changeable. Availability of support, the course the patient's life has taken thus far, and how the patient feels about himself or herself are important factors. Crisis points, such as diagnosis, development of new opportunistic infections, changes in physical ability or appearance, rejection by others, loss of job, and so on, are likely to trigger intense emotional responses. Occasionally, patients will experience diagnosis as a relief, either because they now have an explanation for their symptoms or because they perceive their diagnosis as a way out of a troubled life. Referrals for counseling and support may be indicated.

There are a number of common responses to HIV disease.

DENIAL

Denial is often the first response to learning about one's HIV status or AIDS diagnosis. Denial can be a healthy response because it helps the patient function. Unless the denial is causing the patient to endanger his or her own health or the health of others, it does not need to be confronted. When patients are in denial, they may not be able to process information well. Do not assume that they are comprehending or remembering what you are telling them during this stage. Writing the information down for them to read later, asking them to repeat back to you what you've said, or repeating the information at a later point in time is helpful. Patients are likely to move in and out of denial about different aspects of their disease.

SELF-BLAME

Patients often hold themselves responsible for contracting this disease. Feelings of guilt and shame about their sexual behavior or drug use are likely to surface. For some people with addiction histories, this could trigger a relapse.

In gay patients, internalized homophobia may surface. Some patients experience guilt about the possibility that they may have infected others.

FEAR

Fear is a typical response to diagnosis. Patients are afraid of being sick, dying, suffering, being disfigured, becoming dependent, and losing their mental faculties. Patients also fear rejection, being alone, and not being able to survive economically. Patients are often fearful of entering or maintaining emotional and physical relationships. Parents often have fears about the effect of their disease on their children and about how their orphaned children will be cared for.

ANXIETY

Anxiety about illness progression can rule patients' lives. This may be characterized by obsessive behavior, such as constantly looking for lesions and other physical changes or requesting overly frequent monitoring of T-cells. Patients may fear that minor illnesses are or will turn into life-threatening infections. Sleep disturbances are common.

ANGER

Anger is a typical response to circumstances beyond one's control. Patients may be asking "why me?" and feeling this is unfair. Their anger may be directed at God or the universe. They are also likely to feel angry at themselves, at whoever they believe infected them, at the medical establishment for not being able to cure them, at the disease, at unresponsive bureaucracies, and above all, at their loss of control.

CONTROL

Throughout the course of HIV disease, patients find themselves losing control. This can be control over one's body, disease progression, the ability to act independently, mental status changes, living circumstances, and so on. Diminished control is a major source of frustration and anger for patients. Often, they will lash out at whoever is helping them, because help is another reminder of loss of control. It is useful to maximize patients' sense of control whenever possible. Giving patients choices in their care, involving them in decision making, and respecting their wishes are important means of maximizing patient control. However, sometimes, patients will want things that are unrealistic and that jeopardize their safety, such as being discharged to their homes when they are unable to care for themselves. In these circumstances, the provider or other support person should work with patients to help them understand the reality of their situation. There are times when it may be necessary to override patient desires.

ISOLATION

Patients with HIV often isolate themselves from others. There are many reasons for this. Sometimes isolation can be indicative of an underlying clinical depression. Isolation may be the result of circumstances beyond patients' control, such as job loss; rejection by friends and family members; loss of income; embarrassment about physical changes, such as facial lesions; and physical problems, such as weakness or diarrhea, that inhibit the patient from being able to participate in social functions. At other times, isolation is a choice. Loss of identity and role contributes to patient decisions to isolate. Patients will isolate themselves as a way of defending themselves against anticipated rejection. They may become self-focused and lose interest in others or in activities; they may feel they have nothing positive to contribute to others and prefer to be alone.

LOSS

People with HIV suffer a multitude of losses. These include some of the previously mentioned losses, such as loss of control, identity, role, social networks, physical and mental ability, and a future. For some people, losses may include loss of friends and family to this disease, changes in body image, and the psychological or physical ability to be sexual. Anticipatory grief over impending losses and death is common.

AMBIVALENCE

Patients are often ambivalent about what they want. This is particularly true in the late stages of the disease when a patient may want a way out of suffering but may not really be ready to die. Patients' decisions will be influenced by their level of hope, level of discomfort, and quality of life. Patients may make conflicting requests, which change from day to day. These include requests regarding treatment versus palliative care, life support and DNR (do not resuscitate) issues, and discharge options. It may be necessary to reconfirm patient wishes before acting. Patient ambivalence may be frustrating and time-consuming for you as the provider. Your patience and empathy will make a big difference.

EMPOWERMENT

Some people with HIV are able to use their illness as a means of empowering themselves. For those with a history of addiction, diagnosis may serve as the turning point that starts their recovery process. Speaking out and using this illness as a means of raising awareness or helping prevent others from taking risks gives meaning to some people's lives. Many use their diagnosis to reevaluate their own lives, to heal relationships, and to make choices that change the direction their lives are taking.

SPIRITUALITY

Being faced with a life-threatening illness often leads to an examination of one's spiritual beliefs (see "Spiritual Issues"). Patients may now be coming to terms with the past, making peace with themselves, and reconciling their relationship with God or assessing their spiritual values.

HOPE

Hope is the foundation for maintaining a positive quality of life. Hope provides the basis on which patients can act in their own self-interest—following through on treatment recommendations, entering or continuing a recovery process, achieving a postponed goal, or making amends with estranged family members. Hope is the belief that something is possible and the desire for it to happen. There is no such thing as false hope, even if the hoped-for outcome is highly unlikely. What people hope for is very individual and likely to change. For example, one patient may hope to overcome his or her disease, whereas another may hope for a quick and painless death. Numerous factors, such as how a patient is feeling physically, length of time living with HIV disease, and recent losses or disappointments, influence what a patient hopes for. Sometimes, the hope for something as simple as seeing another Christmas or returning home before dying gives a patient the will to live. It is possible to support hope while reframing the reality of a situation.

Spiritual Issues

Addressing spiritual issues is integral to a holistic approach to HIV care. The impact of spiritual well-being on the overall quality of life and physical healing of a person with AIDS should not be underestimated. Be aware and sensitive to signs that may warrant a referral to a religious or spiritual resource. Religious beliefs held by patients may range from traditional Western Judeo-Christian or Muslim thought to Espiritismo or New Age spirituality. Patients should be encouraged to pursue whatever form of spirituality they choose. Some nontraditional spiritualities offer approaches that are specifically helpful for persons with AIDS. Some patients find spiritual support through 12-step programs or AIDS healing retreats. Whatever the tradition, those living with HIV are confronted by several spiritual issues. Even patients who have not identified themselves as religious often have these concerns. Because these issues are fundamental, they should not be overlooked or avoided by the provider.

Persons living with HIV disease may face the following issues:

- Spirituality and illness
- Concerns about death and suffering
- A desire to be forgiven
- A desire for spiritual support
- Reconciliation with God
- A need for hope

DIFFERING VIEWS OF SPIRITUALITY AND ILLNESS

Providers should be aware of any possible intolerance that may spring from their personal religious beliefs. Imposing one's own spiritual or religious view on the patient can only be counterproductive to the patient-provider relationship. Too often, patients will not return for follow-up care if they feel judged.

If patients hold negative beliefs about themselves they may act in ways that are self-destructive and not follow through on their medical care. This may result in what appears to be noncompliant behavior, such as missing appointments and not taking prescribed medications. It is helpful to listen for questions or statements that reflect a patient's negative self-image.

Persons with HIV disease frequently question why illness has befallen them. They may ask themselves questions such as these:

- Why me?
- Have I been bad?
- Am I being punished?
- What have I done to deserve this?

They may harbor potentially harmful beliefs such as these:

- I am a bad person.
- I deserve to be punished.
- I know that my _____ (promiscuity, homosexuality, drug abuse, etc.) resulted in this.

The basic underlying question for some is this:

- Will God judge me?

Value judgments expressed by providers regarding patients' lifestyles can be detrimental to patients and to the patient-provider relationship. Your value judgments may be used by some patients to reinforce fears about being judged by God.

CONCERNS ABOUT DEATH AND SUFFERING

Patients may have questions about dying or what their experience of death will be. Patients may ask the following:

- Is there life after death, or is death the final chapter?
- Do only good people go to heaven?
- Is death painful? Will I suffer?

Fear of death is often the fear of the unknown. In some patients, fear of the dying process is more overwhelming than fear of death itself. Concerns about suffering, pain, disfigurement, and dependence may arise. For others, worries about being separated from loved ones or fears that no one will remember them after they have died disturb them most. Patients at the end of their lives who have "unfinished business" regarding people in their lives may not be ready to die. However, for some patients, death is not necessarily a negative event.

DESIRE FOR FORGIVENESS

People facing severe illness or death often review their lives. They review both what they have done and what they have left undone. They may regret missed opportunities or abandoned dreams. They may desire to visit a particular place or person. Conversely, they may regret some of their actions. They may desire forgiveness from themselves, from others, or from God.

DESIRE FOR SPIRITUAL SUPPORT

Individuals who have had childhood experiences with religious institutions often feel a need to reconnect with that heritage. This need may also be felt by those who do not have a particular faith heritage. A visit or connection with an established representative from a faith tradition is often helpful.

RECONCILIATION WITH GOD

Patients who feel alienated from their heritage or from God may have a need to reconnect with their spirituality or to reconcile with God. Negative theological messages that patients have internalized, combined with experiences of AIDS discrimination and isolation, may contribute to patient feelings of loneliness, worthlessness, and despair. Gay people, in particular, may be alienated from both their religious institutions and their faith because of negative messages they have heard growing up. Reconciliation with loved ones and God or discovering a new spirituality is often a goal for persons with HIV disease, and they should be supported in this effort.

NEED FOR HOPE

How providers communicate their views of the illness can shape how patients live with this disease. Allowing patients to maintain hope regardless of their medical condition is essential to their spiritual well-being. Hope is a powerful motivator! Presenting HIV disease as an illness some live with for many years before dying allows patients to maintain hope and remain involved in their medical treatment.

NONTRADITIONAL SPIRITUALITY

Providers can reinforce whatever comfort patients are able to derive from their individual beliefs. When making pastoral referrals, providers should inquire as to a patient's spiritual preference.

SOURCES FOR REFERRAL

Encouraging patients to connect with a place of worship or religious leader is often helpful. Also, groups and organizations that offer nontraditional spiritual support are helpful to some patients.

Support Services

Most patients are dealing with myriad issues and concerns because of the complexity of this disease. Many communities offer support services that respond to the holistic needs of patients with HIV disease. Services may be designed to address physical, emotional, mental health, financial, legal, and spiritual concerns. Often, these services are available through specific AIDS service organizations. These services may also be available through churches and other existing service organizations. You or your patient can call the Centers for Disease Control AIDS Clearinghouse (800) 456-5231 to find out how to access AIDS services in your community.

ADVOCACY

Advocacy for a variety of issues, such as legal, financial, housing, and service access, may be available from AIDS service or other community-based organizations.

BUDDIES

Buddies are trained volunteers, usually accessed through AIDS service organizations, who befriend people with HIV disease. These volunteers may provide companionship and support and reduce patient isolation.

CASE MANAGEMENT

Case management is the coordination of service delivery for patients with HIV/AIDS whose multiple needs require referrals to and services from multiple agencies.

Case management should include the following:

- Individual assessment (e.g., physical, mental health, psychosocial needs)
- Needs assessment (e.g., legal, housing, financial, medical needs)
- Service and/or treatment planning
- Linking patient to needed services and/or referrals
- Service implementation and coordination
- Monitoring service provision
- Advocacy to obtain or access services
- Evaluation of care plan
- Documentation of all activities
- Assessment of living situation
- Assessment of patient support

FOOD/MEALS

Some communities have programs that provide meals to people with HIV. This is an excellent way to improve nutrition and reduce isolation simultaneously. Some communities also have programs that offer meal delivery programs to people who are too ill to leave their homes or cook for themselves. Your local AIDS service organization should be able to provide you with details.

PRACTICAL SUPPORTS

Volunteers from AIDS service organizations or churches may be available to provide assistance with odd jobs, homemaking, cooking, baby-sitting, transportation, and other tasks. Your local AIDS service organization will have information.

RESPITE

Respite care may be available from an AIDS service organization, church, visiting nurse association, or hospice.

SUPPORT GROUPS

A variety of support groups are available and are tailored to specific patient needs. This is an inappropriate referral for individuals who indicate that they are not comfortable in group settings. Support groups are often available through AIDS service organizations, churches, mental health agencies, or health care institutions.

ADDITIONAL SUPPORTS

Many communities offer a wealth of services to people with HIV. These can include free haircuts, massage therapy, acupuncture, recreational activities, theater tickets, wellness workshops, and other services. Your local AIDS service organization should be able to provide you and your patients with information.

5

Medical Management

Our understanding of how HIV works and our ability to manage its effect on the individual continues to expand. Several principles of HIV management have emerged to guide practitioners in their care of people with HIV. Early antiretroviral intervention, opportunistic infection prophylaxis, and aggressive diagnosis and treatment are necessary ingredients for providing good care.

Diagnosis and treatment of people with HIV are facilitated by developing an understanding of the major opportunistic infections for which patients are typically at risk. Risks for particular infections often correspond to CD4 cell count; for example, most patients don't develop cytomegalovirus (CMV) retinitis until their CD4 counts fall below 50. A team approach with appropriate subspecialists results in optimal care.

Finally, encouraging patients to participate in their care is likely to result in higher levels of compliance, a more satisfying provider-patient relationship, and improved patient mental and physical well-being.

Pathogenesis of HIV Disease

Early simplistic theories of the pathogenesis of HIV disease suggest that CD4 (helper) lymphocytes are infected by the virus, which results in viral replication and cellular destruction. These events lead to the release of new infectious virions and helper cell depletion. Although this sequence of events occurs, a much more complicated interaction involving the virus, CD4 lymphocytes, cytokines, and other cellular elements takes place.

When an uninfected individual is exposed to HIV virions, the virus binds to CD4 lymphocyte receptors, beginning the long process of HIV infection. Some evidence suggests that Langerhans cells present in mucous membranes may also be infected, which helps to explain sexual transmission. Of infected patients, 50% to 70% experience an acute seroconversion syndrome a few weeks after infection. This coincides with a massive viremia and consists of a mononucleosis-like syndrome with fever, lymphadenopathy, rash, and pharyngitis. These symptoms generally resolve after a few weeks as a brisk antibody response clears the viremia. At this time, HIV serological tests will be positive. Thus begins an asymptomatic period of HIV disease that may last 10 or more years in many individuals or that may be of much shorter duration.

Early studies seem to indicate that the virus is relatively inactive during this clinically latent period. More recent research has shown that HIV is very active in the lymph nodes rather than in the peripheral blood. After initial infection, HIV is located in the lymph node germinal centers' follicular dendritic cells. Here, viral replication takes place with infection of CD4 lymphocytes recruited from the peripheral blood as they migrate through the lymphoid system to fight ongoing infection. Contributing to depletion of CD4 lymphocytes are direct mechanisms such as cell death during viral budding. Indirect mechanisms such as apoptosis (or programmed cell death), superantigen formation, or more recently described autoimmune phenomena also occur. Replication of HIV is at least partially regulated by cytokines, with some facilitating and some suppressing viral replication. As CD4 lymphocytes are destroyed, the body fails to regenerate cells at a pace quick enough to replenish their numbers. Evidence has been presented to show that hematologic function is suppressed, possibly as a direct effect of HIV infection. The sum total of increasing destruction with slowed replacement leads to progressive lowering of the CD4 lymphocyte count. To further complicate this scenario, uninfected CD4 lymphocytes show evidence of defective immune function. A number of mechanisms for this defect have been proposed, but none but none have been proved as yet.

In later stages of HIV infection, the lymph node germinal centers are completely disrupted and large quantities of virus spill into the circulatory system. The body is then unable to continue to control the infection. HIV virion levels in the peripheral blood increase dramatically, creating a heavy viral load. Viral load appears to be correlated with later-stage disease and increased infectiousness. The disruption of the lymph node structure alters the ability of the individual to mount an immune response to a whole host of pathogens. Combined with the depleted CD4 lymphocyte population, these immune system abnormalities lead to the susceptibility of the individual to opportunistic infections.

After an asymptomatic phase, individuals may experience fluctuations in their health. This period, formerly called AIDS-related complex (ARC), is characterized by vague symptoms, including intermittent weakness, fevers, night sweats, localized yeast infections, and other potentially debilitating symptoms. This period is now commonly called symptomatic HIV disease. As the immune system is further depleted, life-threatening illnesses such as *Pneumocystis carinii* pneumonia, toxoplasmosis, *Mycobacterium avium* complex (MAC), and others are likely. Often, patients will experience periods of wellness with only intermittent bouts of illness. Later on in HIV disease, these infections may become more severe and more resistant to treatment and occur concurrently. Wasting syndrome and neurological complications are also common. No two courses of HIV illness are exactly alike. Disease progression is not always linear. Disease management is further complicated by drug interactions and development of resistance to therapies that are used for antiviral, prophylactic, or treatment purposes.

Although management of HIV disease is complex, the following guidelines provide a basis for delivering care to HIV-infected individuals.

CDC AIDS Case Definition

The following AIDS case definition is excerpted from the *Morbidity and Mortality Weekly Report*, December 18, 1992 (Vol. 41, No. RR-17).

REVISED CASE DEFINITION OF AIDS FOR
ADOLESCENTS AND ADULTS, EFFECTIVE 1993

The Centers for Disease Control (CDC) has expanded the AIDS surveillance definition to include all HIV-infected persons who have less than 200 CD4 T-lymphocytes per microliter or a CD4 T-lymphocyte percentage of total lymphocytes of less than 14. This expansion includes the addition of three clinical conditions—pulmonary tuberculosis (TB), recurrent pneumonia, and invasive cervical cancer—and retains the 23 clinical conditions in the AIDS surveillance case definition published in 1987. It is being used by all states for AIDS case reporting effective January 1, 1993 (see Table 5.1).

TABLE 5.1 AIDS Surveillance Case Definition for Adults, 1993

	Clinical Categories		
	A	B	C
	Asymptomatic, PGL, or Acute	Symptomatic,	AIDS Indicator Condition
CD4 Cell Categories	HIV Infection	not A or C Conditions	(1987 definition)
> 500/mm^3 (> 28%)	A1	B1	C1
200-499/mm^3 (14%-28%)	A2	B2	C2
< 200/mm^3 (< 14%)	A3	B3	C3

NOTE: A1, B3, C1, C2, and C3 categories reflect changes in the expanded 1993 definition.

Conditions Included in the 1993 AIDS Surveillance Case Definition.

- Candidiasis of bronchial tubes, trachea, lungs
- Candidiasis, esophageal
- Cervical cancer, invasive
- Coccidioidomycosis, disseminated or extrapulmonary
- Cryptococcosis, extrapulmonary
- Cryptosporidiosis, chronic intestinal (more than 1 month's duration)
- CMV disease (other than liver, spleen, or lymph nodes)
- CMV retinitis (with loss of vision)
- Encephalopathy, HIV related
- Herpes simplex: chronic ulcer(s) (more than 1 month's duration); or bronchitis, pneumonitis, or esophagitis
- Histoplasmosis, disseminated or extrapulmonary
- Isosporiasis, chronic intestinal (more than 1 month's duration)
- Kaposi's sarcoma (KS)
- Lymphoma, Burkitt's (or equivalent term)
- Lymphoma, immunoblastic (or equivalent term)
- Lymphoma, primary, of brain
- MAC or *M. kansasii,* disseminated or extrapulmonary
- *Mycobacterium tuberculosis,* any site (pulmonary or extrapulmonary)
- Mycobacterium, other species or unidentified species, disseminated or extrapulmonary
- *P. carinii* pneumonia
- Pneumonia, recurrent

- Progressive multifocal leukoencephalopathy
- *Salmonella septicemia*, recurrent
- Toxoplasmosis of brain
- Wasting syndrome due to HIV

Category A conditions in Table 5.1 are satisfied when HIV infection is documented and an individual has asymptomatic HIV infection *or* persistent generalized lymphadenopathy *or* acute primary HIV infection with accompanying illness or history of acute HIV infection. Conditions listed in Categories B and C must not have occurred.

Category B consists of symptomatic conditions in HIV-infected adolescent or adults that are not included in clinical Category C and that meet at least one of the following criteria: The conditions are attributed to HIV infection or are indicative of a defect in cell-mediated immunity; *or* the conditions are considered by physicians to have a clinical course or to require management that is complicated by HIV infection.

Category C includes the clinical conditions listed in the AIDS case definition.

Evaluation

I. HISTORY

A. Past medical history: Include surgery, transfusions, transplant, chickenpox or shingles, sexually transmitted diseases (i.e., herpes, syphilis, gonorrhea, warts), hepatitis, exposure to TB and travel history (i.e., tropical diseases, parasites, histoplasmosis, coccidioidomycosis), headache history, use of alternative therapies (herbs, vitamins).

B. Medications and Alternative Therapies

1. Allergies: Include sulfa and Bactrim.

2. Review of systems: Include the appearance of new skin or oral lesions, difficulty in swallowing, sore throat, visual disturbances, new headaches, seizures, intellectual deterioration, memory difficulties, swollen glands, cough, shortness of breath, chest pain, diarrhea, weight loss, fever, sweats, pruritus, sensory disturbances of extremities, penile discharge. Reports of even subtle changes should be noted.

3. Nutritional status

   a) Diet

   b) Food preferences and intolerance

   c) Appetite changes

d) Weight history

e) Eating disorders

f) Previous diet modifications

g) History of megadosing vitamins and minerals

h) Food fads

4. Sexual history

5. Drug/alcohol history (see Chapter 2)

II. PHYSICAL EXAMINATION

A. Record height and weight

B. Perform a detailed physical

1. Skin: Look for KS, warts, psoriasis, seborrhea, fungal infections, syphilitic rashes, bacillary angiomatosis.

2. Fundi: Look for retinitis.

3. Oropharynx: Look for leukoplakia, thrush, KS; assess dental hygiene.

4. Lymph nodes: Look for enlarged nodes.

5. Abdomen: Look for enlarged liver and/or spleen; note absence of spleen.

6. Genitalia: Look for herpetic ulcers, syphilitic lesions, warts, discharge.

7. Rectum: Look for perianal lesions, rectal masses.

8. Nervous system: Look for sensory and motor peripheral neuropathy, early dementia.

III. LABORATORY EVALUATION

A. CD4 count

B. Complete blood count (CBC) + differential + platelets

C. Chemical profile, including liver function tests (LFTs), renal function tests, amylase, etc.

D. Rapid plasma reagin/Venereal Disease Research Laboratory (RPR/VDRL)

1. Initial screening of any and all asymptomatic patients.

2. Patients who received syphilis treatment in the past. Some HIV patients are refractory to standard therapy. The correct therapy for HIV patients has not yet been fully defined. Obtain past documentation of therapy and obtain a current RPR/VDRL.

E. Hepatitis B surface antigen (HBsAg) and hepatitis B core antibody (HBcAb) (see "Immunizations" in this chapter)

F. Culture/smear lesions found at oropharyngeal, skin, genital, or perianal sites

1. Viral culture for herpes

2. Fungal culture/smear for Candida

    3. Bacterial culture for gonorrhea/chlamydia

    4. Dark field for syphilis (if available)

G. Toxoplasmosis titer: Some experts recommend that a baseline toxo titer be drawn to identify patients at risk of developing central nervous system (CNS) toxoplasmosis by reactivation of latent disease.

H. Other viral markers: Currently, the only marker routinely used in therapeutic decision making is the CD4 lymphocyte count. Measurements of a second parameter, such as β2-microglobulin or erythrocyte sedimentation rate (ESR), that is less subject to fluctuation can frequently be helpful in monitoring patients. Studies have shown that the combination of these two values predicts the progression to AIDS better than either value alone.

I. Tuberculin skin testing (PPD—intermediate strength = 5 tuberculin units intradermal)

    1. A tine test is not acceptable. A PPD should be performed unless the patient has a history of TB or a prior positive PPD. A PPD should be performed even if the patient has received BCG (tuberculosis vaccine) in the past. Document previous PPD test results. Anergic patients may have active or dormant TB with a negative PPD.

    2. The criteria for a positive PPD in HIV patients recently have been revised: A positive test has traditionally been considered to be an induration of more than 10 mm. However, in HIV patients an induration of more than 5 mm is considered positive, even if the patient had received BCG.

    3. An anergy screen (Candida and/or mumps intradermal) is also recommended by the CDC.

Treatment

I. GENERAL

A. Provide information on HIV disease (see Chapter 1).

B. Refer patient to specialty physicians as necessary.

C. Promptly report AIDS cases to state or local health departments as required by law, using the recently revised CDC surveillance case definition for AIDS. Call local or state health departments for assistance.

II. NUTRITIONAL COUNSELING

A. Multivitamin prescription

B. Develop a nutritional care plan with a registered dietitian if available. Set up an individualized meal plan based on the following:

    1. Calorie/protein needs

2. Food intolerance
3. Weight loss (more than 10% premorbid weight)
4. Anorexia
5. Nausea and/or vomiting
6. Diarrhea
7. Constipation
8. Taste alterations
9. Fever
10. Dry and/or sore mouth
11. Sore throat and dysphagia
12. Need for nutritional supplements
13. Need for help in arranging nutrition support economically (e.g., food banks, soup kitchens)

C. Follow-up nutritional care should be included with each clinic visit.

III. IMMUNIZATIONS

A. Give pneumococcal vaccine (Pneumovax) once; repeat every 5 years.

B. Give influenza vaccine in October every year.

C. Adult tetanus-diphtheria (Td) toxoid should be given every 10 years. Initial series should be given if the patient has never been immunized.

D. Measles, mumps, rubella (MMR) vaccines can be administered as recommended for non-HIV patients when CD4 count is more than 500. For patients with CD4 count of less than 500, consult an infectious disease specialist.

E. Oral polio vaccine (OPV) should not be given to HIV patients. Due to reports of polio disease in the immunosuppressed patient, inactivated polio vaccine (IPV) has been suggested as an alternative. In addition, the administration of OPV to infants is not recommended if there is an HIV patient in the same household.

F. Hepatitis B vaccine (Heptavax, Recombivax)

1. HBsAg seronegative intravenous drug users or seronegative sexually active patients who continue to engage in high-risk activity should be vaccinated. Counsel HBsAg-positive patients regarding transmissibility and immunize close contacts.

2. The exact immunization protocol for HIV patients has not yet been defined. HIV patients may not respond to the primary hepatitis B vaccination. The vaccination doses and schedule recommended by the CDC for dialysis and immunocompromised patients are currently applied to HIV patients— dosage: 40 μg at 0, 1, and 6 months in the deltoid muscle.

3. Follow-up after primary hepatitis B immunization: Testing for immunity (i.e., HBsAg of more than 10 mIU/ml) is recommended for HIV patients within 1 to 6 months after vaccination. Even though only a small number of nonre-

sponders will develop immunity after one or two boosters, revaccination should be attempted. Booster dosage: 40 μg in the deltoid muscle. Retest for immunity (i.e., HBsAg of more than 10 mIU/ml) 1 to 6 months later.

NOTE: Patients who do not develop immunity after a primary vaccination course and two boosters are unlikely to respond to revaccinations.

4. Patients who responded to hepatitis B vaccine and patients who give a history of having received hepatitis B vaccine should be tested for immunity (i.e., HBsAg of more than 10 mIU/ml) semiannually. Administer a 40 microgram booster in the deltoid muscle as needed and follow response.

5. Travelers requiring immunization: Consult an infectious disease specialist, a physician experienced in HIV care, or a travel clinic.

IV. INTERPRETATION OF CD4 COUNT

NOTE: Critical treatment decisions should not be based on a single determination of the CD4 count because wide fluctuations have been documented. Each patient should have repeat CD4 counts performed at the same laboratory at the same time of day to avoid interlaboratory and diurnal variations. CD4 counts also fluctuate during acute illness. Test results indicating a change in treatment course should be repeated for verification.

CD4 count more than 700	Repeat in 6 months.
CD4 count 500-700	Repeat in 3 months.
CD4 count 200-500	See "Antiviral Therapy" in this chapter.
CD4 count less than 200	See "Antiviral Therapy." In addition, *Pneumocystis carinii* pneumonia (PCP) prophylaxis should be recommended.

NOTE: For a CD4 count of less than 500, follow-up counts should be obtained every 2 to 3 months or until the CD4 count falls below 200. An increase in the frequency of opportunistic infections has been noted for patients with a CD4 count of less than 50, and some consultants advise following CD4 counts and counseling the patient regarding signs and symptoms of opportunistic infections (see Table 5.2).

Be aware that zidovudine (ZDV, brand name Retrovir) treatment will cause a transient increase in CD4 counts for up to 6 months. Once treatment with ZDV has been initiated, it should not be discontinued if subsequent CD4 counts are more than 500.

V. ANTIRETROVIRAL THERAPY

NOTE: At the IX International Conference on AIDS, held in June 1993, many questions were raised about usage of antiviral medications—ZDV, didanosine, and zalcitabine. The standard of practice was to start ZDV in asymptomatic

TABLE 5.2 Relationship Between CD4 Counts and Disease Progression

CD4 = 300 to 400	Usually few or no symptoms • Some thrush • Herpes zoster • Bacterial infections (pneumonia, sinusitus) • Hairy leukoplakia • Kaposi's sarcoma/lymphoma • Tuberculosis	
CD4 ≤ 200	*Pneumocystis carinii* pneumonia (PCP), thrush	
CD4 ≤ 100	• Severe cytomegalovirus (CMV) • *Mycobacterium avium* complex (MAC) • Toxoplasmosis • Severe diarrheal disease • Cryptosporidiosis • Adrenalitis • Wasting syndrome	Observations • Condition can deteriorate rapidly Subtle presentations • Coexistence of multiple infections • More adverse reactions to medications • Poor nutrition may play a role
CD4 ≤ 50	• Increased incidence of all HIV disease, especially CMV, MAC • Increased risk of death from all HIV-related diseases	

patients when their CD4 count drops below 500. This standard was developed on the basis of results of an early study of ZDV (ACTG 019). A larger, longer study (Concorde trial) presented at the meeting, convincingly showed that such early use of ZDV may be of no clinical benefit. In addition, the utility of CD4 counts as a marker of treatment success or failure was questioned.

A National Institutes of Health (NIH) consensus panel convened soon after the conference had made the following preliminary recommendations.

A. NIH recommendations for patients who have never before received antiretroviral therapy

1. For patients without symptoms whose CD4 cell counts are above or equal to 500/mm³, the panel recommends continued observation and clinical and immunologic monitoring (measurement of CD4 cell counts) every 6 months.

2. For patients without symptoms whose CD4 cell counts are 200 to 500/mm³ and who are stable over time, the panel recommends consideration of the following two options:

   a) Initiation of antiretroviral therapy

   b) Continued observation and monitoring for clinical or laboratory evidence of deterioration, at which point antiretroviral therapy should be initiated.

3. For patients with CD4 cell counts of 200 to 500/mm³ who present with symptoms related to HIV disease, the panel recommends starting antiretroviral therapy.

B. NIH recommendations for choosing initial antiretroviral therapy

1. Use ZDV as first-line therapy in patients who have received no prior anti-retroviral therapy. The recommended dose is 600 mg per day in divided doses.

2. The recommendation to initiate therapy with ZDV applies to patients with or without symptoms, with CD4 cell counts of 200 to 500/mm^3 or below 200/mm^3, or to patients with severe symptomatic HIV disease or AIDS regardless of their CD4 cell counts.

3. Combination therapy with ZDV and didanosine or ZDV and zalcitabine may also be considered, although clinical trials have not conclusively demonstrated clinical benefit to date.

C. NIH recommendations for changing initial therapy in patients tolerating an initial antiretroviral therapy

1. For patients tolerating initial therapy, who appear to be stable with CD4 cell counts above 300/mm^3, the panel recommends continuing ZDV.

2. For patients who have CD4 cell counts below 300/mm^3, the panel recommends consideration of two options:

   a) Continuing ZDV

   b) Changing to didanosine

NOTE: The panel notes that the strongest data supporting a change in therapy to didanosine were seen in patients who had been on ZDV for 4 months or longer (medium duration of 13 months prior to ZDV).

D. NIH recommendations for ZDV intolerance or ZDV failure

1. For patients with CD4 cell counts of 200 to 500/mm^3 and 50 to 200/mm^3 who are intolerant of ZDV, the panel recommends switching to didanosine mono-therapy. For ZDV-intolerant patients with CD4 cell counts of less than 50/mm^3, the panel recommends switching to didanosine or zalcitabine mono-therapy. Another option includes discontinuing antiretroviral therapy.

2. For patients with CD4 cell counts of 200 to 500/mm^3 and 50 to 200/mm^3 who show signs of clinical progression, the panel recommends initiating an alternative antiretroviral regimen. Options include monotherapy—for example, with didanosine—or initiation of combination therapy by adding a second agent, either didanosine or zalcitabine.

3. For patients with CD4 cell counts above 500/mm^3 who are taking ZDV but experience intolerance, the panel recommends discontinuation of therapy.

NOTE: Providers who care daily for large numbers of HIV-infected patients are not surprised by this controversy. Adoption of a healthy lifestyle, close medical follow-up, opportunistic infection prophylaxis, and early intervention when symptomatic have long been the keys to success in treating HIV. Above all, a close patient-physician partnership with open discussion of treatment options and participation by the patient in therapeutic decision making is required.

E. ZDV

1. Indications for therapy
   a) CD4 count of less than 500
   b) Unexplained thrombocytopenia
   c) The patient has AIDS, regardless of CD4 count
   d) Lymphocytic interstitial pneumonitis
2. Relative contraindications for therapy
   a) Hemoglobin less than 8.0 g/dL
   b) Absolute neutrophil count of less than 1,000
3. Dosage
   a) ZDV 100 mg every 4 hours × 5 times a day, while awake
      or
   b) ZDV 200 mg every 8 hours

NOTE: Patients with concomitant liver and kidney diseases require modified doses. For the use of ZDV in pregnancy, see Chapter 7.

4. Laboratory monitoring while on ZDV
   a) CBC + differential + platelets—prior to treatment, after 2 weeks, then monthly. If stable, then may be done every 2 or 3 months.
   b) LFTs, blood urea nitrogen (BUN), creatinine—prior to treatment, after 2 weeks, then every 3 months.
   c) Creatinine phosphokinase (CPK): Every 6 months

NOTE: Monitor patients with cytopenia more frequently. Use of other medications that affect bone marrow function or the presence of liver or renal disease also require closer monitoring.

5. Complications of ZDV therapy
   a) Minor: headaches, insomnia, and nausea. These usually subside with continued treatment and are not usually of such severity to stop treatment.
      (1) Headaches can be managed with acetaminophen or nonsteroidal anti-inflammatory medications.
      (2) Nausea can be managed symptomatically.
      (3) Insomnia can be managed with mild sedatives.
   b) Major: anemia, neutropenia, and myositis
      (1) Anemia (hemoglobin < 7.5 g/dL): Manage with transfusions and/or recombinant erythropoietin. The dose of ZDV can be temporarily reduced to 100 mg every 8 hours. If applicable, consider didanosine or ZDV and/or zalcitabine
      (2) Neutropenia
         (a) Absolute neutrophil count (ANC) less than 750 cells/mm^3: ½ dose ZDV

(b) ANC less than 500 mm^3: Discontinue ZDV until the count recovers, following which therapy can be restarted at a lower dosage with close monitoring. Use of G-CSF or GM-CSF (granulocyte stimulating factors) can be considered if necessary. If applicable, consider didanosine or ZDV/zalcitabine.

(c) Myositis: ZDV should be discontinued and muscle enzymes (CPK, aldolase) monitored. If applicable, consider didanosine.

F. Didanosine

1. Indications

   a) Intolerance of ZDV

   b) Clinical/laboratory deterioration while on ZDV therapy

   c) Patients with advanced HIV infection who have received prolonged prior ZDV therapy

2. Dosage (*always taken on an empty stomach*)

   a) Didanosine chewable tablets

   > $\geq$ 60 kg = two 100-mg tablets twice a day (bid)
   > < 60 kg = one 100-mg tablet *and*
   >   one 25-mg tablet bid

   b) Didanosine buffered powder for oral solution

   > $\geq$ 60 kg = one 250-mg packet bid
   > < 60 kg = one 167-mg packet bid

3. Laboratory monitoring while on didanosine

   a) CBC + differential + platelets—prior to treatment, after 2 weeks, then monthly. If stable, may then be done every 2 to 3 months.

   b) LFTs, BUN, uric acid, creatinine, amylase—prior to treatment, after 2 weeks, then monthly

NOTE: Monitor patients with cytopenia more frequently. Use of other medications that affect bone marrow function or the presence of liver or renal disease also require closer monitoring.

4. Complications

   a) Minor: diarrhea, headache, and abnormal laboratory values (see package insert). If diarrhea and headache are severe, reduce dose or stop therapy.

   b) Major: pancreatitis, peripheral neuropathy

      (1) Pancreatitis ranges from mild to fatal. Increased serum amylase is a nonspecific sign. If amylase increases to 2× baseline, didanosine should be discontinued and then restarted at a lower dose (100 mg bid). Patients with a history of pancreatitis, alcohol abuse, hypertriglyceridemia, or renal disease are at greater risk for pancreatitis and should be followed more closely.

      (2) Peripheral neuropathy is characterized by distal numbness, tingling, or pain in the feet or hands. Didanosine should be held until

neuropathy resolves. Patients may be able to tolerate resumption at a reduced dose.

G. Zalcitabine (Hivid)

1. Indications for therapy: In combination with ZDV, zalcitabine is indicated for the treatment of patients with advanced HIV infection who have demonstrated significant clinical or immunologic deterioration. (Zalcitabine has recently been shown to be of benefit when used alone as well.)

2. Dosage: zalcitabine 0.750 mg orally every 8 hours with ZDV 200 mg orally every 8 hours

NOTE: Dosage should be lowered in the presence of renal or hepatic impairment

3. Laboratory monitoring while on zalcitabine: CBC, chemistry profile, amylase, triglycerides—prior to treatment, after 2 weeks, then monthly

NOTE: Monitor patients with cytopenia more frequently. Use of other medications that affect bone marrow function or the presence of liver or renal disease also require closer monitoring.

4. Complications of zalcitabine

a) Peripheral neuropathy: Stop zalcitabine until symptoms resolve and then restart at 50% dosage (i.e., zalcitabine 0.375 mg orally every 8 hours).

b) Pancreatitis: Stop therapy at first signs and/or symptoms of pancreatitis, with asymptomatic rising amylase, or during treatment with other medications that may cause pancreatitis (e.g., intravenous [IV] pentamidine). Restart zalcitabine only if pancreatitis has been ruled out. If pancreatitis occurs during therapy, zalcitabine should be permanently discontinued.

c) Oral ulcerations

H. d4T (stavudine, Zerit): Stavudine is a nucleoside reverse transcriptase inhibitor similar to ZDV. In May 1994 a Food and Drug Administration (FDA) Antiviral Advisory Panel recommended that d4T be approved for use in a subset of HIV-infected patients. Indications for therapy and effective dosing range have yet to be established. Preliminary data suggest that adverse effects will include anemia, peripheral neuropathy, and possible pancreatitis. For more information call 1-800-842-8036.

I. Alternative regimens

1. Recent studies have shown that patients who take acyclovir in combination with ZDV have higher survival rates than those who take ZDV alone. Recommended dosage is 800 mg by mouth (po) four times a day (qid).

2. Patients who cannot tolerate ZDV, didanosine, or zalcitabine: Investigational protocols are availabl (see Chapter 8).

Asymptomatic patients with normal CD4 counts (> 700): Investigational protocols are available (see Chapter 8).

VI. *PNEUMOCYSTIS CARINII* PNEUMONIA (PCP) PROPHYLAXIS

A. Definitions

1. Primary prophylaxis: treatment that is given to prevent the first episode of PCP

2. Secondary prophylaxis: treatment that is given after the first episode of PCP to prevent additional episodes.

B. Indications for primary prophylaxis

1. Patients with clinically defined AIDS who have not had PCP

2. Patients with laboratory-defined AIDS (CD4 count < 200)

3. Consider with CD4 nearing 200 and symptoms (e.g., thrush)

C. Pretherapy screening

1. Chest X-ray optional

2. Evaluation for TB (see *M. tuberculosis* under "Pulmonary Manifestations" in the "Common Symptoms" section of this chapter).

3. Allergies: Specifically inquire about sulfa and trimethoprim/sulfamethoxazole (Bactrim, Septra).

D. Prophylactic regimens

1. Preferred regimen: Use trimethoprim/sulfamethoxazole, double strength, one tablet every day three times a week (Monday, Wednesday, Friday).

2. Alternative regimens: aerosolized pentamidine 300 mg every 4 weeks. Treatment can be administered at home or in clinics. Patients who develop cough and bronchospasm may benefit from pretreatment with an aerosolized bronchodilator 10 minutes prior to the aerosolized pentamidine. This treatment is suitable for patients who are allergic to sulfas, are pregnant, or have bone marrow suppression.

   or

3. Dapsone: dosage range 100 mg po every week or 100 mg po every day (most effective dose not known). Suitable for patients who are allergic to sulfas and intolerant of aerosol treatments. G6PD (glucose-6-phosphate dehydrogenase) screening is recommended prior to starting dapsone.

VII. *MYCOBACTERIUM AVIUM* COMPLEX (MAC) PROPHYLAXIS: RIFABUTIN (MYCOBUTIN)

A. Indications: Disseminated MAC occurs most commonly when CD4 count is less than 100. FDA-approved indication for starting rifabutin prophylaxis is a CD4 count less than 200.

NOTE: The use of rifabutin is still controversial.

B. Dosage: Rifabutin 150-mg tablets—2 tablets every day

C. Laboratory monitoring: Blood cultures for MAC (Dupont Isolator) should be drawn prior to initiation of treatment to rule out active disseminated MAC. Prophylaxis can be begun prior to obtaining culture results. LFTs should also be monitored.

D. Complications of rifabutin: orange urine, rash, neutropenia, LFT abnormalities, interaction with other drugs, gastrointestinal (GI) intolerance, iritis, pseudo-jaundice, drug interactions

E. Drug interactions: Rifabutin alters hepatic metabolism of many drugs.

Common Medical Problems Encountered in HIV Disease

I. COMMON SYMPTOMS

A. Fever with a low CD4 count

1. Evaluation

a) History and physical: Particular attention is paid to common sites of opportunistic infections—for example, pulmonary (PCP, TB), CNS (cryptococcosis, toxoplasmosis), GI (infectious diarrhea), cardiac (endocarditis in injection drug user), or drug-induced fever.

b) Laboratory: Include a CBC, a urinalysis and culture, a chest X-ray (CXR), blood cultures for bacteria and MAC, serum cryptococcal antigen, liver enzymes for hepatitis, and amylase and sputum (if obtainable) for routine culture and TB stains or cultures.

c) Follow-up: Patients who are unreliable or in whom follow-up is not ensured should be considered for hospitalization for their diagnostic evaluation.

2. Nonspecific treatment: As adjunctive therapy or until a specific etiology is found, the following can be used:

a) Acetaminophen 650 mg or aspirin 650 mg po every 4 hours around the clock. If needed, these may be alternated every 2 hours. As an alternative, use ibuprofen 400 to 600 mg po every 4 hours.

b) Tepid or sponge baths can be used for unresponsive fever.

c) Fluid replacement should be encouraged.

B. Diarrhea: See Diarrhea under "GI Manifestation" in this section.

1. Evaluation

a) Laboratory: See Diarrhea under "GI Manifestation" in this section.

b) Specialty referral: If the above evaluation is unrevealing, a gastroenterologist should be consulted for endoscopy and possible biopsy of the colonic and/or duodenal mucosa to identify other possible pathogens.

2. Follow-up

   a) Patients should be hospitalized if they become dehydrated or appear toxic or if the above studies identify a source of diarrhea that requires hospitalization for effective treatment.

   b) Patients who are unreliable or in whom follow-up is not ensured should be considered for hospitalization for their diagnostic evaluation.

3. Nonspecific treatment: As adjunctive therapy or until a specific etiology is found, the following can be used:

   a) Discontinue foods/supplements that may aggravate diarrhea.

   b) For mild diarrhea: kaolin/pectin (Kaopectate) 60 to 120 cc po after each bowel movement

   c) For more severe diarrhea:

      (1) Diphenoxylate/atropine (Lomotil) 1 to 2 tabs po qid as needed
         or

      (2) Loperamide (Imodium) 4 mg po to start, then 2 mg po after each diarrheal bowel movement with a maximum of 16 mg per day
         or

      (3) Somatostatin: 50 μg subcutaneously three times a day (tid), which may be increased to 500 μg SQ tid.
         or

      (4) Deodorized tincture of opium: 2 drops in glass of water, bid

C. Nausea/vomiting

1. Multiple types of infections, KS, and various medications may cause nausea and vomiting.

   a) Laboratory: LFTs, amylase, and lipase should be checked. Consider serum cortisol level. If persistent, an upper GI series should be obtained.

   b) Specialty referral: If persistent, GI consult should be obtained for endoscopy with possible biopsies of esophagus/duodenal mucosa.

2. Nonspecific treatment: The following can be used:

   a) Liquid or low-residue diets with smaller, more frequent meals are often better tolerated. Pay particular attention to adequate hydration and nutrition.

   b) Medications as follows:

      (1) Prochlorperazine (Compazine) 5 to 10 mg po qid
         or

      (2) Prochlorperazine 25-mg rectal suppository bid
         or

      (3) Promethazine (Phenergan) 25 to 50 mg po every 4 to 6 hours
         or

      (4) Haloperidol (Haldol) 0.5 to 5 mg po bid
         or

  (5) Metoclopramide (Reglan) 10 mg po tid after meals

c) Nonapproved therapies

  (1) Dronabinol (Marinol) 5 mg/m^2 to 15 mg/m^2, 2 to 6 times per day. *Caution*—can create drowsiness and anxiety and be addictive.

  (2) Ondansetron hydrochloride (Zofran) dosage and interval not established for this use. *Caution*—can cause diarrhea and headache.

D. Neurological symptoms

1. New onset of seizures or focal deficits: Hospitalize for computerized axial tomography (CAT) or magnetic resonance imaging (MRI) scan and possible cerebrospinal fluid (CSF) examination.

2. Headache (new onset or change in severity and/or duration of chronic headache): If the history and physical is nonfocal and the patient recently began ZDV, treatment may be symptomatic. Headache associated with ZDV usually resolves spontaneously within 6 to 8 weeks of initiating treatment.

   a) If the CD4 count is more than 350, opportunistic infections are unlikely. If the history and physical is nonfocal, then reassurance and observation are acceptable.

   b) If the CD4 count is less than 200, opportunistic infections are very possible. If the patient is afebrile with a nonfocal examination, a serum cryptococcal antigen test should be obtained. If the patient is febrile or the headache history is unusual or suspicious, the patient should be hospitalized for cerebral imaging studies and lumbar puncture. If the serum cryptococcal antigen test is negative and the patient remains afebrile but the headaches persist, outpatient cerebral imaging studies should be obtained.

   c) If the CD4 count is between 200 and 350, patients should be approached as if the CD4 count is less than 200.

E. Visual changes: Loss of visual field or acuity: These visual changes may be caused by CMV retinitis, which, when untreated, can lead rapidly to blindness. Other infections (e.g., toxoplasmosis, TB) are much less likely causes. Patients should have an immediate dilated fundoscopic examination. If this is not possible or the examiner is unsure of the findings, patients should have immediate evaluation by an ophthalmologist. If CMV retinitis is diagnosed, patient should be hospitalized for IV ganciclovir or IV foscarnet in consultation with an infectious disease specialist.

F. Respiratory problems: Dyspnea

1. Patients should have a thorough history and physical, paying particular attention to the pulmonary examination.

2. Laboratory: A CXR is mandatory. Presence of specific abnormalities on the X-ray should prompt a search for a specific pathogen. Desaturation of hemoglobin detected by digital oxymetry with exercise may be valuable. Evaluation of arterial blood gases may be indicated.

3. Differential diagnosis

    a) PCP: A history of low-grade fevers, dry cough, onset of symptoms over weeks in a patient with CD4 less than 200 suggests pneumocystis pneumonia. See Infections—PCP—under "Pulmonary Manifestations" in this section.

    b) Bacterial pneumonia: A history of high fever, productive cough (purulent sputum), characteristic sputum gram stain, and lobar/bronchopneumonia pattern on CXR should suggest bacterial pneumonia. See Infections—Bacterial pneumonia—under "Pulmonary Manifestions" in this section.

    c) Tuberculosis: TB should be considered in all HIV patients with respiratory disease. See *M. tuberculosis* under "Pulmonary Manifestations" in this section.

G. Weight loss ·

    1. Any infection or neoplasm can present with weight loss as a manifestation. Particular attention is paid to GI disease (e.g., diarrhea) or difficulty with eating due to dental disease. MAC is a frequent cause of weight loss. A diagnosis of idiopathic AIDS wasting syndrome should not be made until treatable causes are eliminated. Cytokines have been postulated as possible mediators.

    2. Laboratory: Besides routine blood work and symptom-directed testing, a blood culture for MAC should be obtained.

    3. Nonspecific treatment: As adjunctive therapy, or until a specific etiology is found, the following can be used:

        a) Nutritional supplements

        b) Appetite stimulants

            (1) Dronabinol 2.5 mg po bid prior to lunch and supper

            (2) Megestrol (Megace) 80 mg po qid, may be increased to 160 mg po qid

        c) Tumor necrosis factor (TNF) inhibitor: pentoxifylline (Trental) 400 mg po tid with meals. Elevated triglycerides may be used as an indirect, nonprecise marker of increased TNF.

II. PULMONARY MANIFESTATIONS

A. Infections

    1. PCP

        a) Clinical presentation: PCP is the most common pathogen in HIV patients. Clinically, PCP presents with slow, progressively increasing symptoms (median duration before diagnosis is 28 days). Most prominent is dyspnea, initially on exertion only. Fever is present in two thirds of patients and nonproductive cough in one half. Extrapulmonary infection is rare but does occur, including the middle ear, mastoid, retina, liver/spleen, bone marrow, and lymph nodes. Physical findings are usually few. Laboratory findings are also few, although an isolated elevation of lactate dehydrogenase (LDH) with a negative CXR may be a clue. Arterial blood gases usually show hypoxemia but may not correlate well with severity of the infection as judged by CXR. Pulmonary function testing most commonly demonstrates a decrease in diffusing capacity. The most common radiological finding is a diffuse interstitial or perihilar pattern with peripheral sparing, although virtually any pattern can be seen, including pneumothorax, cavitation, lobar consolidation, and a normal chest film in 5% to 10% of cases. Pleural effusions are uncommon with PCP alone.

b) Diagnosis: Clinical (X-ray) diagnosis is possible, but microbiological diagnosis is preferred. Sensitivities of preferred diagnostic techniques are as follows:

Bronchoalveolar lavage (BAL)	85-97%
Transbronchial biopsy (TBB)	97%
Combined BAL and TBB	near 100%
Sputum induction	55-79%

Gallium scanning and pulmonary function testing are nonspecific indicators of disease and should be reserved for situations in which you suspect infection but have a negative CXR.

c) Treatment: Patients can be treated without hospitalization for presumptively diagnosed mild PCP if they meet the following criteria:

(1) CXR is negative or with early infiltrates.

(2) Alveolar-arterial gradient is less than 30 mm Hg.

(3) PO_2 is more than 70 mm Hg.

NOTE: Before undertaking outpatient therapy, be sure that close clinical and laboratory monitoring and follow-up are guaranteed. Ideally, this should include every-other-day visits by the patient's provider or a visiting nurse.

(a) Trimethoprim 15 to 20 mg/kg per day with sulfamethoxazole 75 to 100 mg/kg per day for 21 days divided into four equal doses each day.

NOTE: This is given as double-strength tablets containing trimethoprim 160 mg and sulfamethoxazole 800 mg each.

(b) For sulfa allergic patients, dapsone (Dapsone) 100 mg po every day for 21 days with trimethoprim (Proloprim, Trimpex) 20 mg/kg body weight every day for 21 days.

(c) Atovaquone (Mepron) 750 mg po tid for 21 days. Must be taken with fatty food. Side effects commonly include rash, nausea, and diarrhea. Vomiting is seen less frequently.

(d) Clindamycin 600 mg po qid and primaquine 15 mg po every day for 21 days.

      (e) For treatment failures, trimetrexate (Neutrexan) can be used in a
          closely monitored, inpatient setting.

2. *M. tuberculosis*

NOTE: TB presents a major public health as well as clinical problem. Among
HIV-infected people who have a positive PPD, the rate of developing active TB
disease is 7% per year. In addition, the emergence of multidrug resistant TB
(MDRTB) is on the rise due to inadequate treatment. Assistance is generally
available through state health departments for patients who need direct observed
therapy (DOT) or who need help obtaining medication.

    a) Clinical: TB can occur early in the course of HIV disease. Its presentation
       may differ depending on the severity of HIV immune system damage. In
       relatively healthy HIV patients, TB is clinically similar to TB in non-HIV
       patients. Symptoms will be very nonspecific, consisting of fever, cough,
       weight loss, and possibly night sweats. CXR in these patients is often more
       typical, revealing upper-lobe infiltrates, occasionally with cavitation. Un-
       fortunately, nonspecific infiltrates are also common, requiring that TB be
       part of the differential diagnosis of any pulmonary infiltrate.

        In later stages of HIV disease, TB can present in an atypical manner.
       Extrapulmonary disease is a very common presentation for these patients.
       Most common extrapulmonary sites include lymphatic system, GI tract,
       genitourinary tract, and bone marrow. Other sites, including the CNS, may
       be involved. Most of these patients also have some pulmonary involvement
       at the time of their presentation. CXRs tend to be more nonspecific with
       lower-lobe infiltrates, miliary fever and noncavitary disease being most
       common.

    b) Diagnosis: All patients with pulmonary infiltrates should be tested to
       eliminate TB as a possible etiology, using sputum smear for acid-fast stain
       and sputum culture for Mycobacterium. Patients with suspicious infil-
       trates and no diagnosis may require BAL to increase diagnostic yield. CXR
       may be negative in 20% of patients. Tuberculin skin testing (PPD) by
       Mantoux method may be helpful but is limited by a high degree of anergy
       in HIV patients. For HIV patients, 5 mm of induration is considered to be
       a positive tuberculin test. Report to the state health department.

    c) Treatment: Patients with acid-fast bacilli found on smear should be treated
       for TB until their culture results are finalized. In general, treatment of TB
       in HIV patients is very effective, providing that the medical regimen is
       completed. Adverse drug reactions are much more frequent in HIV pa-
       tients using antituberculous medications, so clinical and laboratory moni-
       toring of therapy is essential.

      (1) Pulmonary TB: Isoniazid (INH) 300 mg po every day and rifampin
         (Rifadin) 600 mg po every day (450 mg if < 50 kg) and pyrazinamide
         (Pyrazinamide) 20 to 30 mg/kg body weight each day divided tid or
         qid (maximum 2 gm/day) and ethambutol for the first 2 months of
         therapy and pyridoxine (vitamin B6) 10 to 25 mg po every day with

INH to prevent neuropathy. INH and rifampin should be continued indefinitely or for 6 months after cultures turn negative.

(2) CNS or disseminated disease: Same regimen as above and ethambutol (Myambutol) 15 to 25 mg/kg po every day (maximum 2.5 gm/day). INH, rifampin, and ethambutol should be continued for a total of 9 months of therapy or for 6 months after cultures turn negative. Periodic ophthalmologic examination should be provided for patients taking ethambutol.

d) Prophylactic therapy of PPD-positive asymptomatic patients: Obtain a chest X-ray. Duration of treatment has not been clearly defined. Some specialists suggest treatment for life, whereas others suggest treatment for at least 12 months. Treatment should not be withheld if patient is over 35 years old.

(1) INH 300 mg po every day (unsupervised) or INH 15 mg/kg po (maximum 900 mg) twice a week (supervised). Schedule follow-up visits for monitoring INH toxicity.

(2) Pyridoxine 10 mg every day.

e) Prophylactic therapy of PPD-negative asymptomatic patients: Contacts with active cases of TB should receive prophylaxis. Prior to the initiation of therapy, obtain a CXR. Use the regimen detailed above.

3. Bacterial pneumonia: A history of high fever, productive cough (purulent sputum), characteristic sputum gram stain, and lobar/bronchopneumonia pattern on CXR should suggest bacterial pneumonia (usually pneumococcus or *Hemophilus influenzae*). Patients with a normal arterial blood gas who do not appear toxic or in severe distress may be considered for treatment with oral antibiotics in an outpatient setting. Outpatient treatment should be considered only in very reliable patients who can be followed closely.

III. SYPHILIS

A. RPR-positive asymptomatic patient: Confirm with fluorescent treponemal anti-body-absorption test (FTA-ABS). False positive syphilis serology (RPR/VDRL-positive but FTA-ABS-negative) has been well described in injection drug users, patients with lupus and infective endocarditis, and HIV patients. If FTA-ABS is positive: Treat patient according to stage. Report positive serology to state health department.

B. Clinically suspected syphilis with negative or unknown serology: HIV patients may have atypical manifestations or an accelerated course. CNS syphilis may develop in young patients and should be included in the differential diagnosis of neurological disease in HIV patients. There have been reports of HIV patients with biopsy-proven syphilis with negative serology. Treat as outlined next.

C. Treatment: The CDC has not changed recommendations for therapy of HIV patients with syphilis.

1. Primary, secondary, and early latent syphilis
   a) Benzathine penicillin G 2.4 million units intramuscularly (IM) × one dose
      or
   b) Tetracycline 500 mg po qid × 2 weeks

NOTE: Some specialists advise CSF examination and/or treatment for neurosyphilis for HIV patients regardless of the stage, even if there are no signs or symptoms of neurosyphilis. Tetracycline is not recommended in pregnancy.

2. Neurosyphilis
   a) Aqueous crystalline penicillin G 2 million units IV every 4 hours × 10 days
      or
   b) Aqueous procaine penicillin G 2.4 million units IM every day × 10 days
      and with either regimen
   c) Probenecid 500 mg po qid × 10 days

NOTE: Some specialists recommend additional treatment after the above regimens with benzathine penicillin G 2.4 million units IM every week × 3 weeks.

3. Late latent syphilis, cardiovascular syphilis, and tertiary syphilis
   a) Benzathine penicillin G 2.4 million units IM every week × 3 weeks
      or
   b) Tetracycline 500 mg po qid × 4 weeks

D. Follow-up after treatment: VDRL should be repeated at 3, 6, and 12 months. Reevaluate the patient for treatment failure, reinfection, or neurosyphilis if
   1. VDRL titer does not decrease appropriately (two-dilution decrease by 3 months for primary syphilis or by 6 months for secondary syphilis).
   2. VDRL titer increases by two dilutions or more.

IV. ORAL MANIFESTATIONS

A. Hairy leukoplakia
   1. Clinical presentation: Lesions appear as asymptomatic, whitish thickening of the oral mucosa that can be as small as a few millimeters or involve very large areas. The etiology is felt to be Epstein-Barr virus-induced hyperplasia.
   2. Diagnosis: Diagnosis is usually clinical, although if the practitioner is unsure or the lesion appears suspicious, referral to an oral surgeon for biopsy is indicated.
   3. Treatment: Rx is generally not necessary. Lesions may respond to acyclovir 800 mg po 5 times a day.

B. Candidiasis
   1. Clinical presentations: Oral candidiasis can present as four different types of lesions:

a) Atrophic: Usually, a chronic, red erythematous lesion on the palate and dorsum of the tongue.

b) Pseudomembranous (thrush): Creamy white plaques anywhere in the oral cavity that bleed when removed by scraping.

c) Chronic hyperplastic: Red and white lesions anywhere in the oral cavity that are not removed by scraping.

d) Angular cheilitis: Redness and fissuring that occur unilaterally or bilaterally at the angles of the mouth that may occur alone or with other forms of candidiasis.

For patients with dysphagia and oral candidiasis see Dysphagia Due to Esophagitis under "GI Manifestations" in this section.

2. Diagnosis: Usually made on the basis of the clinical appearance. Potassium hydroxide smears or culture on appropriate fungal media may be helpful. Occasionally, biopsy of the lesions is needed for diagnosis, especially for the atrophic or hyperplastic lesions.

3. Treatment

a) For mild to moderate cases

(1) Nystatin oral suspension (Mycostatin) (100,000 units/cc): 5 cc swish and swallow qid × 14 days

or

(2) Nystatin oral pastilles (200,000 units): 1 or 2 pastilles dissolved slowly in the mouth 5 times a day × 14 days

or

(3) Clotrimazole troches (Mycelex) (10 mg): 1 troche dissolved slowly in the mouth 5 times a day × 14 days

b) For severe or resistant cases

(1) Ketoconazole (Nizoral) 200 mg po every day × 14 days. This may need to be increased to 400 mg po every day.

or

(2) Fluconazole (Diflucan) 200 mg po the first day, then 100 mg po every day × 14 days

or

(3) Itraconazole (Sporonox) 200 mg po the first day, then 100 mg po every day × 14 days

or

(4) Amphotericin B troches 200 mg po qid × 14 days or parenteral amphotericin B 20 to 30 mg IV three times a week

c) Prophylaxis for recurrent cases: Most patients will require continuous prophylaxis.

(1) Nystatin oral suspension (100,000 units/cc): 5 cc swish and swallow qid

or

    (2) Nystatin oral pastilles or clotrimazole troches: 1 dissolved slowly in the mouth tid

       If these prophylaxis regimens fail

    (3) Fluconazole 200 mg po the first day, then 100 mg po every day

       or

    (4) Itraconazole 200 mg po the first day, then 100 mg po every day

C. Periodontal disease (gingivitis, periodontitis)

  1. Periodontal disease may be a cause of weight loss. Nutritional intake should be monitored very closely.

  2. Prevention: Meticulous attention to good oral hygiene is essential, including regular toothbrushing and use of dental floss. Early referral to routine dental care is advisable.

  3. Treatment: These patients must be referred for dental care. Local debridement is the key to successful therapy. Pending dentist's care, the following medication may be helpful:

    a) Chlorhexidine oral rinse (Peridex) (0.12%): 15 cc swished around gums for 30 seconds then expectorated bid after toothbrushing.

D. Oral ulcers

  1. Clinical presentation: Multiple organisms can cause oral ulcerations. In general, treatment should be based on specific identification of the etiologic agent.

    a) Herpesvirus (herpes simplex, varicella-zoster, CMV) present as grouped vesicles on an erythematous base. Frequently, the vesicles are ruptured and a nonspecific ulceration is the only remnant.

    b) Recurrent aphthous ulcers (RAU) are fairly common. Three types are described, which can all be painful and persist for several weeks.

      (1) Minor RAU: 0.5-cm to 1.0-cm solitary lesions, well circumscribed with erythematous margins

      (2) Herpetiform RAU: Clusters of 1- to 2-mm ulcers on the soft palate or oropharynx

      (3) Major RAU: Large necrotic ulcers 2 to 4 cm in size

  2. Diagnosis

    a) Diagnosis of herpesvirus may be made clinically, although confirmation with viral culture is preferred.

    b) Diagnosis of RAU is made by exclusion. Viral culture should be obtained to eliminate other possible etiologies. Suspected major RAU should always be initially referred to an oral surgeon for a biopsy to rule out malignancy as a diagnostic consideration.

    c) Ulcerations that are suspicious or resistant to treatment should be biopsied.

  3. Nonspecific treatment: Nutritional/fluid intake must be closely monitored.

a) Diphenhydramine suspension (Benadryl) (5 mg/cc) mixed with an equal amount of kaolin/pectin (mixed by pharmacist) applied directly to lesions on an as-needed basis.

or

b) Viscous lidocaine (Xylocaine) 2% applied directly to lesions on an as-needed basis. This should not be swallowed, to avoid inhibition of the patient's gag reflex with possible aspiration.

4. Specific treatment

a) Herpes simplex

(1) Acyclovir (Zovirax) 200 mg po 5 times a day until ulcers resolve

(2) Prophylaxis for recurrent ulcers: acyclovir 400 mg po bid indefinitely

b) Varicella-zoster: Mild/moderate outbreak: acyclovir 800 mg po 5 times a day until all lesions have crusted

c) RAU: Use fluocinonide ointment (Lidex) (0.05%) or triamcinolone acetonide ointment (Aristocort) (0.1%) mixed with 50% orabase applied to ulcers 5 or 6 times a day until resolved.

(1) For multiple ulcers or difficulty with applying above medication: Use dexamethasone elixir (Decadron) 0.5 mg per cc as a mouth rinse, then expectorated, 5 or 6 times a day until resolved.

(2) For large lesions unresponsive to topical therapy, consider prednisone (Deltasone) 40 to 60 mg per day po × 7 to 10 days.

d) For severe or unresponsive ulcers of the types listed above, consider hospitalization for IV medication.

e) Thalidomide has been used successfully but should be used only in consultation with an infectious disease specialist. Further information is available through the National Hansen's Disease Center in Carville, LA (pharmacy: 1-504-642-4762; treatment investigational new drugs [INDs] for aphthous stomatitis: 1-504-346-5785).

E. Oral warts (human papillomavirus [HPV])

1. Diagnosis: clinical appearance, although biopsy may be necessary

2. Treatment: referral to an oral surgeon for removal

V. GI MANIFESTATIONS

A. Dysphagia/odynophagia due to esophagitis

1. Clinical presentation: Any patient who presents with pain or difficulty swallowing should be evaluated for possible esophageal infection. The most common pathogen, either alone or in combination with other organisms, is Candida. Other common pathogens are herpes simplex and CMV.

2. Diagnosis: Diagnosis can initially be made empirically. A diagnosis of infectious esophagitis is sufficient to classify the patient as having AIDS.

3. Treatment

   a) Candida esophagitis

      (1) Mild/moderate disease

         (a) Use ketoconazole 200 mg po every day × 14 to 21 days.

           or

         (b) Use fluconazole 200 mg po the first day, then 100 mg po every day × 13 to 20 days

NOTE: The above regimens should be followed by prophylaxis with one of the oral prophylaxis regimens. See Candidiasis—Prophylaxis— under "Oral Manifestations" in this section.

      (2) Severe or refractory cases

         (a) Hospitalize for IV therapy.

         (b) Evaluate for resistant candidiasis.

   b) CMV (biopsy proven): Hospitalize for IV ganciclovir or foscarnet.

   c) Herpes simplex (biopsy proven): Hospitalize for IV therapy.

B. Diarrhea (enterocolitis)

   1. Clinical presentation: Any patient presenting with diarrhea of more than a few days' duration should be evaluated for possible enteric pathology (see Figure 5.1). The following is a differential diagnosis:

Acute	Chronic
Shigella sp.	*Cryptosporidium* sp.
Salmonella sp.	Microsporidium
Campylobacter sp.	*Isospora belli*
Aeromonas sp.	*Mycobacterium avium*
Clostridium difficile	Cytomegalovirus
Giardia lamblia	Kaposi's sarcoma
Entamoeba histolytica	Lymphoma
Other parasites	HIV enteropathy

   2. Diagnosis: Diagnosis of these conditions is based on stool examinations. The following tests are suggested to diagnose the most common pathogens: stool for gram stain and acid-fast stain

   3. Routine stool culture

      a) *Clostridium difficile* toxin

      b) Ova and parasites × 3

      c) Examination for *Cryptosporidium* sp., *Isospora belli*, and Microsporidium must be ordered separately.

      If these tests fail to yield a pathogen and the diarrhea is persistent, referral to a GI specialist is advised.

   4. Nonspecific treatment: See Diarrhea under "Common Symptoms" in this chapter.

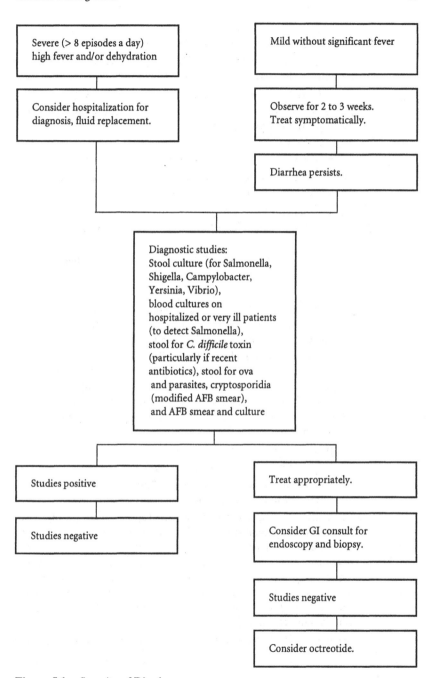

Figure 5.1.   Severity of Diarrhea

5. Specific treatment

   a) *Aeromonas* sp.: Use ciprofloxacin (Cipro) 500 mg po bid × 7 days.

   b) Amebiasis (*Entamoeba histolytica*): Use metronidazole (Flagyl) 500 mg po tid × 10 days followed by iodoquinol (Yodoxin) 650 mg po tid × 20 days

   c) *Campylobacter* sp.: Use ciprofloxacin 500 mg po bid × 7 days.

   d) *C. difficile*: Use metronidazole 250 mg po TID × 7 days (preferred due to the high cost of vancomycin)

      or

      Use vancomycin (Vancocin) 125 mg po qid × 7 days

   e) *Cryptosporidium* sp.: Refer to infectious disease specialist. Several reports document success with paromomycin or azithromycin.

   f) CMV: Hospitalize for IV ganciclovir or foscarnet.

   g) *Giardia lamblia*: Use metronidazole 250 mg po tid × 7 days.

      or

      Use quinacrine hydrochloride (Atabrine) 100 mg po tid after meals × 5 days.

   h) *I. belli*

      (1) Acute treatment: Use trimethoprim/sulfamethoxazole DS (Bactrim DS, Septra DS) po qid × 10 days, then trimethoprim/sulfamethoxazole DS po bid × 14 days. Prophylax indefinitely: Use trimethoprim/sulfamethoxazole DS po three times a week.

      (2) If allergic or intolerant to Bactrim or Sulfa, use pyrimethamine (Daraprim) 25 mg with folinic acid 5 mg po every day. Prophylax indefinitely: Use pyrimethamine 25 mg with folinic acid 5 mg po every day.

   i) KS: See Kaposi's sarcoma under "Neoplastic Disorders" in this section. Consult an oncology specialist.

   j) Lymphoma: Consult an oncology specialist.

   k) Microsporidium: Consult an infectious disease specialist.

   l) *Mycobacterium avium intracellulare*: See "*Mycobacterium avium* Complex" in this section. Consult an infectious disease specialist.

   m) *Salmonella* sp. (nontyphoidal): If the patient appears toxic or septic, he or she should be hospitalized for evaluation of possible septicemia. If the patient does not appear toxic or septic, obtain blood cultures prior to treatment and initiate an outpatient oral regimen. If blood cultures subsequently grow Salmonella, hospitalization for intravenous antibiotics may be necessary. Use ciprofloxacin (Cipro) 500 mg po bid × 14 days. After 14 days, the patient should be reevaluated. Prolonged therapy or chronic suppression may be necessary.

   n) *Shigella* sp.: Use trimethoprim/sulfamethoxazole DS (Bactrim DS, Septra DS) po bid × 7 days.

6. HIV enteropathy: This condition should be diagnosed only when an exhaustive search for a pathogen fails. Treatment: Monitor nutritional/fluid intake.

   a) Use the nonspecific therapies listed earlier.

   b) Opiates such as paregoric may be necessary to control the diarrhea.

   c) Consider empirical trials of antibiotics.

   d) Consider a trial of investigational protocols in consultation with infectious disease or GI specialists.

C. Jaundice/hepatomegaly

1. Clinical manifestations: The following are the major causes of liver/biliary disease in HIV patients. Although abnormal LFTs are not uncommon in these patients, symptomatic disease is uncommon.

Hepatic Parenchymal Disease

Mycobacterium avium complex	Hepatitis C
Medications (especially sulfa)	Histoplasmosis
Cryptococcus	Coccidiomycosis
Lymphoma	*Microsporidium* sp.
Kaposi's sarcoma	Peliosis hepatis
Hepatitis B	Bacillary angiomatosis
Biliary disease	Papillary stenosis
Sclerosing cholangitis	
(due to CMV, Cryptosporidium)	
Lymphoma	

2. Diagnosis: Ultrasound and LFTs are used to differentiate intrahepatic from extrahepatic (biliary) disease. Hepatitis serologies are ordered where appropriate. A therapeutic trial of withholding potentially hepatotoxic medications might be useful when the etiology of hepatic parenchymal disease is unclear. Liver biopsy for hepatic parenchymal disease is reserved for symptomatic disease that is suspected of having treatable etiology. Most infectious causes are systemic with other means of diagnosis available. Endoscopic retrograde cholangiopancreatiography (ERCP) is usually used to further define the cause of extrahepatic obstruction.

3. Treatment: Treatment should be directed toward the specific infectious agent or neoplasm that has been identified. For hepatic parenchymal disease, potentially hepatotoxic medications should be discontinued.

D. Proctitis

1. Clinical presentation: Proctitis usually presents as frequent small-volume stools, left lower quadrant or suprapubic pain, tenesmus, and painful defecation. Frequently, a purulent discharge or small volume of bright red blood will be present. The differential diagnosis listed later includes a number of sexually transmitted diseases. In addition, the usual causes of inflammatory bowel disease may be present (i.e., ulcerative colitis or Crohn's colitis). Colorectal neoplasms are not uncommon in these patients and should always be excluded in undiagnosed patients.

2. Diagnosis

Differential Diagnosis

Neisseria gonorrhoeae	Syphilis
Chlamydia trachomatis	Human papillomavirus
Herpes simplex	Cytomegalovirus

Obtain appropriate rectal cultures for gonorrhea, herpes, and chlamydia. In addition, obtain a rectal swab for a gram stain and acid-fast stain. Order a serological test for syphilis. If the preceding tests fail to reveal the diagnosis, consider empirical treatment. If the diagnosis is still unclear, referral to a GI specialist for sigmoidoscopic culture and biopsy is indicated.

3. Treatment

a) Gonorrhea (diagnosis by culture or smear)

(1) Use ceftriaxone (Rocephin) 250 mg IM as a single dose with doxycycline (Vibramycin) 100 mg po bid × 7 days.

or

(2) Use ofloxacin (Floxin) 400 mg po as a single dose (do not use if pregnant) with doxycycline 100 mg po bid × 7 days.

NOTE: In pregnancy, substitute for doxycycline: Use erythromycin (E-Mycin) 500 mg po qid × 7 days.

b) Chlamydia

(1) Use doxycycline (Vibramycin) 100 mg po bid × 7 days.

(2) In pregnancy, substitute for doxycycline: Use erythromycin (E-Mycin) 500 mg po qid × 7 days.

c) Herpes

(1) Use acyclovir (Zovirax) 200 mg po 5 times a day until resolved. If no response within 48 hours, use acyclovir (Zovirax) 400 mg po 5 times a day until resolved.

d) HPV: Refer to an ano-rectal surgeon for treatment.

NOTE: For severe disease, empirical treatment pending test results is acceptable using the following regimen. Be sure to obtain all cultures/smears prior to treatment.

Use ceftriaxone (Rocephin) 250 mg IM as a single dose or ofloxacin (Floxin) 400 mg po as a single dose and doxycycline (Vibramycin) 100 mg po bid × 7 days and acyclovir (Zovirax) 400 mg po 5 times a day.

VI. DERMATOLOGIC MANIFESTATIONS

A. Bacterial infections

1. Staphylococcus: The most common bacterial pathogen is *Staphylococcus aureus*, usually presenting as folliculitis, bullous impetigo, ecthyma, cellulitis,

or hidradenitis suppurativa-like plaques. Infections respond to the usual antistaphylococcal regimens.

2. Epithelioid (bacillary) angiomatosis: Epithelioid angiomatosis is closely related to cat-scratch disease, presenting as cutaneous pyogenic granulomas, although visceral involvement occurs. Diagnosis is usually by biopsy. Cutaneous infection responds to erythromycin, rifampin, or gentamycin.

3. Syphilis: See Syphilis under "Common Medical Problems" in this chapter.

B. Viral infections

1. Herpes virus infections

a) Mucocutaneous herpes simplex (Types 1 or 2)

(1) Clinical presentation: Lesions appear as grouped vesicles on an erythematous base. Vesicles may be ruptured and appear as shallow ulcerations. Purulent exudate usually is indicative of secondary infection of the lesions.

(2) Diagnosis: Diagnosis is made clinically by appearance, although viral culture may be obtained in questionable cases.

(3) Treatment

(a) General measures

(i) Keep lesions clean and dry. Gentle cleansing with mild soap and water is recommended for lesions in areas subject to contamination (ano-genital). A blow-dryer on a low setting may help to keep lesions dry.

(ii) Analgesics should be provided as needed.

(iii) Loose fitting clothing may help provide comfort.

(b) Medications for an acute attack

(i) Mild/moderate: Use acyclovir (Zovirax) 200-400 mg po 5 times a day for 10 days.

(ii) Severe: Hospitalize for IV acyclovir (Zovirax).

(c) Prophylaxis for frequent recurrences or indolent infections

(i) Use acyclovir (Zovirax) 400 mg po bid indefinitely.

or

(ii) Use acyclovir (Zovirax) 200 mg po tid indefinitely.

(d) Acyclovir-resistant virus: Consult infectious disease specialist for foscarnet (Foscavir) IV.

b) Varicella-zoster virus (VZV) infection (shingles or chickenpox)

(1) Clinical presentation: Primary varicella (chickenpox) infection in HIV patients is usually severe and frequently life threatening. Herpes zoster infection (shingles) appears as vesicles on an erythematous base in a dermatomal distribution. In HIV patients, multidermatomal involvement is common. Usually, the rash is preceded by a few days of radicular pain/burning/pruritus. The ophthalmic division of the tri-

geminal nerve may be involved, resulting in corneal involvement. Ophthalmology should be consulted if there is involvement of the tip of the nose.

(2) Diagnosis: Diagnosis is usually made on the basis of history of prodromal symptoms and the presence of a typical rash. Viral culture can be obtained if the diagnosis is in question. Treatment should be initiated pending culture results.

(3) Treatment

(a) General measures: See herpes simplex virus infections covered under "Oral Manifestations" in this section.

(b) Medications

(i) Opthalmic zoster, disseminated zoster, or severe dermatomal zoster: Hospitalize for acyclovir (Zovirax) IV.

(ii) Mild/moderate dermatomal zoster: Use acyclovir (Zovirax) 800 mg po 5 times a day until all lesions have crusted.

(c) Patients should be instructed to drink at least four 8-ounce glasses of water a day to avoid renal toxicity.

NOTE: Patients with primary varicella should be managed in consultation with an infectious disease specialist due to the potentially life-threatening nature of this illness.

(4) VZV exposure (chickenpox or shingles): The following steps should be taken for HIV patients intimately exposed to VZV (e.g., family contact of chickenpox) with no prior history of infection with VZV (chickenpox or zoster) or a negative serum antibody titer:

(a) Within 96 hours of exposure, consult with an infectious disease specialist for possible use of zoster immunoglobulin (ZIG).

(b) After more than 96 hours after exposure, consult with an infectious disease specialist as soon as possible. At appearance of the first lesion begin acyclovir (Zovirax) 800 mg po 5 times a day.

2. Molluscum contagiosum

a) Clinical presentation: Lesions numbering from one to hundreds usually appear on the face, with a predilection for the eyelids, in the genital area, or on the trunk. They usually appear as umbilicated, pearly papules, 2 to 5 mm in size, with cheesy core. Occasionally, they will exceed 1 cm.

b) Diagnosis: Diagnosis is usually clinical. Biopsy is necessary only if the diagnosis is not apparent.

c) Treatment: Lesions are treated only for cosmetic reasons. If small in number, lesions can be opened with removal of the cheesy core. Other destructive modalities, such as cryotherapy, laser therapy, or surgical removal, can be used. Retin-A 0.05% cream can be applied nightly to help prevent new lesions. This should not be applied to the ano-genital areas or eyelids. *Retin-A should not be used by pregnant women.*

3. HPV (*Condyloma acuminata*, venereal warts)

a) Clinical presentation: Lesions are usually soft, fleshy, single to multiple, papillary, or sessile from 1 mm to many cms in size. They may number from one to many and usually occur in an ano-genital or oral location.

b) Diagnosis: Diagnosis is usually made by appearance. Biopsy can be used if malignancy is suspected. Vinegar can be applied topically to the area to be examined to better visualize lesions.

c) Treatment

(1) Podophyllin 20% in tincture of benzoin is applied to the lesions and allowed to dry. Intact skin is masked with petrolatum. The area is thoroughly washed after 4 hours. Treatment can be repeated weekly until lesions resolve. *Podophyllin should not be used for oral, meatal, cervical, or ano-rectal warts. It should also not be used for pregnant women or for extensive lesions.*

or

(2) Destructive modalities, such as cryosurgery, laser surgery, or electro-cautery, can be used.

NOTE: Women with HPV infection need especially close monitoring with Pap smears and/or colposcopy for detection of cervical neoplasia.

C. Fungal infections

a) Tinea or Candida: Superficial tinea or Candida infections are very common in HIV patients. Infections can be resistant to therapy, which usually consists of topical or oral antifungal agents.

b) Cryptococcosis, histoplasmosis, sporotrichosis, and blastomycosis are four fungal infections that can present with dermatologic manifestations. Skin lesions with these fungi are an indication to search for systemic infection, which will require systemic treatment. Biopsy is usually required for diagnosis.

D. Noninfectious dermatologic conditions

1. Xerosis/ichthyosis

a) Clinical presentation: Lesions present as dryness with a fine scale, usually located on the anterior lower legs but may be widespread. Pruritus is frequent with skin breakdown in severe cases.

b) Diagnosis: Diagnosis is based on clinical appearance.

c) Treatment

(1) Avoid frequent bathing, especially with deodorant soaps.

(2) Apply moisturizing lotion or cream to skin when bathing and in the evening (e.g., Eucerin, Lubriderm).

(3) Severe cases

    (a) Hydrocortisone ointment 1% or 2.5% applied tid

    or

    (b) Triamcinolone ointment (Aristocort, Kenalog) 0.025% applied tid

2. Seborrheic dermatitis

  a) Clinical presentation: Seborrheic dermatitis occurs in up to half of all HIV patients. Lesions are mildly erythematous with a yellowish, greasy scale. The most common locations are the face (eyebrows, lashes, nasolabial folds, in and around the ears), scalp, and center of the chest (especially if hairy). Less common lesions occur in the axilla and groin. Scalp and trunk lesions tend to be pruritic.

  b) Diagnosis: Diagnosis is based on clinical appearance and tests to eliminate other causes (e.g., fungal smears and cultures).

  c) Treatment

    (1) Mild cases

      (a) Scalp

        (i) Selenium sulfide shampoo (Selsun Blue) on a regular basis

        or

        (ii) Tar shampoo (e.g., Zetar Shampoo) on a regular basis

        in addition if needed

        (iii) Triamcinolone solution 0.1% applied bid

      (b) Other areas

        (i) Acute therapy

          (aa) Hydrocortisone cream 1% or 2.5% applied bid to qid

          or

          (bb) Desonide cream (Tridesilon) 0.05% applied bid

          add to either if needed

          (cc) Ketoconazole cream (Nizoral) 2% applied every day

        (ii) Maintenance therapy is usually required: Use regimens for acute therapy but a frequency of every day to twice a week.

        (iii) Severe or refractory cases: Reevaluate for another diagnosis. Consider dermatology referral. Try more potent topical steroids in areas other than the face or genitalia. *In addition*

          (aa) Ketoconazole (Nizoral) 200 mg po every day for 2 to 4 weeks

          or

          (bb) Fluconazole (Diflucan) 200 mg po the first day, then 100 mg po every day for 2 to 4 weeks

3. Psoriasis: Psoriasis in HIV patients is usually similar to that in non-HIV patients. Diagnosis and treatment are also similar.

4. Reiter's syndrome: Reiter's syndrome is fairly common in HIV patients. The syndrome presents as a systemic disease, including arthritis as the primary manifestation, urethritis, conjunctivitis, circinate balanitis, and keratoderma blenorrhagia. Diagnosis and treatment do not differ from the non-HIV population.

5. Hypersensitivity reactions

   a) Drug eruptions: Drug eruptions are very common and are seen in up to half of HIV patients who take trimethoprim/sulfamethoxazole (Bactrim, Septra). Other drugs, such as zidovudine (ZDV) and acyclovir (Zovirax), rarely cause a drug eruption. The most common lesion is a diffuse maculopapular rash. Other reactions include urticaria, exfoliative erythroderma, fixed drug eruption, erythema multiform, and toxic epidermal neurolysis.

   b) Insect bite reactions: HIV patients frequently have more severe responses to insect bites. Lesions appear as papular urticaria. Most common offenders are scabies mites, fleas, and mosquitoes. Diagnosis is clinical or uses scrapings/biopsy for scabies. Treatment is standard for these conditions.

6. Eosinophilic folliculitis

   a) Clinical presentation: Lesions appear as pruritic folliculitis, similar to staphloccocal folliculitis. The eruption is chronic with a waxing and waning course. Lesions may be edematous papules up to 1 cm with a tiny central pustule. They appear as a few to many lesions scattered on the trunk, head, and neck.

   b) Diagnosis: Lesions are culture-negative for *S. aureus.* Biopsy reveals an eosinophilic infiltrate. There is no response to antibiotic therapy.

   c) Treatment

      (1) Antihistamines as needed for pruritus
         and

      (2) Medium- to high-potency topical steroid creams

      (3) If no response, try psoralen ultraviolet A light (PUVA) therapy.

7. Photosensitivity: Lesions appear as erythematous patches and plaques located on sun-exposed areas. Lesions may be prevented by use of sunblocks.

8. Pruritic papular eruptions of unknown etiology

   a) Diagnosis: Skin biopsy and cultures are often needed.

   b) Treatment

      (1) Empirical treatment for Staphylococcus
         then, if no response

      (2) Medium- to high-potency topical steroid creams
         and

      (3) Antihistamines as needed for pruritus

(4) An ointment formulated as follows, applied bid, has been found to give symptomatic relief. In a 240-g jar mix equal amounts of the following:

> Triamcinolone 0.1%
> Urea 10% USP
> Phenol 1/4%
> Menthol 1/4%

VII. NEOPLASTIC DISORDERS

A. Kaposi's sarcoma (KS)

1. Clinical presentation: Varies from the finding of a few skin lesions to a debilitating process manifest as innumerable, large, disseminated mucutaneous lesions involving lymph nodes and visceral organs, most notably the GI tract, mouth, and lungs. Organ compression with internal bleeding can occur.

2. Diagnosis: Diagnosis is based on clinical impression or biopsy. Skin exam should attempt to quantify the lesions (0, < 10, 10-50, > 50). Tumor-related edema of the legs, genitalia, and periorbital regions should be noted.

3. Clinical staging: There is no fully accepted clinical staging system. Limited disease is considered as having fewer than 25 lesions and no evident pulmonary or GI involvement. Those with more advanced lesions and/or profound immune deficiencies are considered to have extensive disease.

4. Treatment: In general, treatment of KS should be comanaged with an oncologist. Limited disease can often be treated with local therapies, whereas more extensive disease requires a more aggressive approach. Presence of a few KS lesions does not mandate therapy. Local measures that have been proved effective in control of KS lesions of the skin include surgical excision, radiation therapy, application of liquid nitrogen, and intralesional injection of dilute concentrations of the antineoplastic agent vinblastine. Alpha-interferon is an agent useful in patients with limited disease. It has little activity in patients with CD4 counts of less than 200. Alpha-interferon should be comanaged with infectious disease or oncology specialists because side effects may be significant and less toxic alternatives should be considered. The combination of ZDV and interferon appears to have not only an antineoplastic effect but augmented antiretroviral activity as well. Extensive KS has been effectively treated with conventional chemotherapy. The intent of this therapy is purely palliative. Complete responses are rarely seen, and partial response rates have ranged from 25% to 75%.

B. Non-Hodgkin's lymphoma (NHL)

1. Clinical presentation: Spectrum of NHL in AIDS is distinctly different than lymphomas seen in the nonimmunocompromised patient and is almost exclusively of B-cell origin. High-grade lymphomas (Burkitt's and immunoblastic sarcoma) are seen with much higher frequency and are generally disseminated at presentation. Intermediate-grade lymphomas (large-cell) tend to

behave more aggressively. Most common sites of extranodal involvement include the GI tract, CNS, liver, and bone marrow. The CNS can be involved as lymphomatous meningitis or epidural masses. However, there has been an increased incidence of primary CNS B-cell lymphoma presenting as a space-occupying lesion that must be distinguished from toxoplasmosis.

2. Treatment: Involves multiagent chemotherapy. For primary CNS lymphoma, treatment involves combinations of radiation, steroids, and chemotherapy, which have shown limited success.

VIII. NEUROLOGICAL MANIFESTATIONS

A. Central nervous system (CNS)

1. AIDS dementia complex (ADC)

a) Clinical presentation: ADC is very common and increases in frequency with advancing disease. It is usually absent before symptomatic HIV disease develops. However, it may be the presenting problem. Clinically, ADC is characterized by a triad of cognitive, motor, and behavioral dysfunction. Early on, there are signs of inattention, poor concentration, forgetfulness, slowed movements, clumsiness, ataxia, apathy, and social withdrawal. Late in the course, there is global dementia, paraplegia, and mutism. In general, symptoms evolve over a period of months. Motor dysfunction usually develops after cognitive dysfunction.

b) Diagnosis: ADC must be differentiated from depressive disorders (pseudo-dementia). The presence of asymmetrical, focal deficits would be atypical and raise concerns about mass lesions or progressive multifocal leuk-oencephalopathy (PML). CAT or MRI scans and spinal fluid analysis are recommended to rule out other potential etiologies. Cerebral atrophy is the only finding on CAT scanning. MRI will show increased signal intensity. Neuropsychological testing will usually show abnormalities early in the course of dementia.

c) Treatment: ZDV should be started because it has been shown to improve symptoms in some patients (if not already receiving the drug).

2. Opportunistic infections

a) *Toxoplasma gondii*

(1) Clinical presentation: Toxoplasma, a protozoan, is the most common cause of intracerebral mass lesions. Infection is usually acquired from raw meat and contact with cat feces. Active infection usually represents reactivation of latent infection. Fifty percent of all adults have evidence of prior infection. Up to 30% of HIV patients with a positive baseline serology will eventually develop toxoplasma encephalitis. Frequently, symptoms are mild, vague, or nonspecific. A constant, dull headache is the most common complaint. Mild to moderate alterations in mental status are common. Thirty percent of patients have focal findings on examination; 15% to 30% have seizures (the most com-

mon infectious cause of seizures in HIV patients). Patients may have weeks to months of subtle symptoms prior to presentation.

(2) Diagnosis: CAT scanning may demonstrate single or more commonly multiple, ring-enhancing lesions in the basal ganglia or corticomedullary junction. Double-dose contrast CAT studies have an improved yield. However, CAT scan may miss lesions; MRI scanning is more sensitive, usually detecting multiple lesions. CSF examination (after CAT scan only) in cases in which diagnosis is uncertain is usually fairly normal with normal glucose, slight protein elevation, and a mild mononuclear pleocytosis. Serological studies are unreliable for acute diagnosis of toxoplasmosis, although a negative titer weighs against the diagnosis.

(3) Treatment: Patients are hospitalized due to the severity of their illness and the need to monitor therapy. Pyrimethamine/sulfadiazine or clindamycin are used under the guidance of an infectious disease specialist. Most patients respond to therapy within 10 days. CAT scans show improvement in 3 to 6 weeks. Suppression must be continued throughout the patient's life to prevent reactivation of disease. There are no current recommendations for prophylaxis, although a number of regimens are under investigation.

(4) Treatment failures: Consult infectious disease specialist for possible atovaquone (Mepron) or azithromycin (Zithromax) treatment.

b) *Cryptococcus neoformans*

(1) Clinical presentation: Cryptococcus is a yeast. It is the most common fungal infection of the CNS. In HIV patients, 10% will develop cryptococcosis, although it is a more common infection in injection drug users or black individuals. Initial pulmonary infection is usually asymptomatic. Presentation is as a slowly progressive meningitis. Onset is subtle with nonspecific complaints, such as malaise, fever, headache, nausea, or vomiting, which may be present for a month before diagnosis. Subtle personality changes may be noted. Occasionally, no CNS signs or symptoms are present. Seizures are rare. Disseminated disease (lungs, bone marrow, liver, prostate, skin, or bone) occurs in 60% of patients with cryptococcosis.

(2) Diagnosis: CAT scan is usually nondiagnostic, although a focal lesion (cryptococcoma) may rarely be seen. CSF examination is mandatory. This usually reveals increased pressure, minimal lymphocytic pleocytosis (5 cells/cc), elevated protein (in 50%), and decreased glucose (in 30%). Specific diagnosis is made by (a) CSF india ink stain (+ in 75%), (b) CSF cryptococcal antigen (> in 90%), and (c) CSF culture (+ in 100%). Serum cryptococcal antigen is positive in 95% of cases, often earlier than CSF antigen. Positive serum antigen tests in the absence of clear-cut symptoms should prompt a search for disseminated cryptococcosis.

NOTE: All HIV patients with fever and systemic symptoms of unclear etiology should have a serum cryptococcal antigen performed as part of their fever workup, even in the absence of CNS signs/symptoms.

(3) Treatment

    (a) Acute disease: Treatment with amphotericin-B or fluconazole (Diflucan) is generally initiated in the hospital in consultation with an infectious disease specialist.

    (b) Maintenance: Fluconazole (Diflucan) is the preferred agent because it can be administered orally. Dose is 200 mg every day.

    (c) Prophylaxis: There are no current recommendations for prophylaxis, although a number of regimens are under investigation.

c) Aseptic meningitis

    (1) Clinical presentation: Aseptic meningitis is frequently a manifestation of initial seroconversion. Symptoms may be acute/self-limited or chronic/recurrent. Presentation is with a headache, fever, meningismus, and usually no focal neurological signs, although cranial nerve palsies may occur.

    (2) Diagnosis: Diagnosis must rule out more serious etiologies. CSF examination may show only mononuclear pleocytosis and elevated opening pressure. Scans are normal.

    (3) Treatment: Symptomatic only.

d) Progressive multifocal leukoencephalopathy (PML)

    (1) Clinical presentation: PML is a demyelinating disease of cerebral white matter caused by papovavirus JC. Presentation is subacute or as a chronic illness. Personality/cognitive changes occur early, with focal findings seen later, such as hemiparesis, hemianopia, or ataxia with increasing dementia. Progressive deterioration is rapid, with death usually occurring in 3 or 4 months. Ten percent of cases involve only the brain stem or cerebellum. The symptoms may be difficult to distinguish from those of AIDS dementia complex if focal findings are mild.

    (2) Diagnosis: CAT or MRI scans may show focal or diffuse lesions in the white matter without contrast enhancement or mass effect. Frequently, scans are normal and diagnosis is clinical or at autopsy.

    (3) Treatment: No effective treatment is available.

e) Encephalitis: Encephalitis of any etiology other than toxoplasmosis is rare but may be caused by viruses (herpes simplex, herpes zoster, cytomegalovirus, HIV) and fungi (candidiasis, aspergillosis, coccidiomycosis, mucormycosis).

3. Neoplastic diseases: See "Neoplastic Disorders" in this section.

B. Spinal cord disease

  1. Vacuolar myelopathy

    a) Clinical presentation: Vacuolar myelopathy is most commonly accompanied by dementia and thus felt to be part of ADC. It can, however, occur alone. It is felt to be a direct infection of the spinal cord by HIV. Onset is subacute and progressive with a painless gait disturbance, ataxia, and spasticity. Bladder and bowel problems occur after the onset of the gait disturbance. Sensory deficits are less common.

    b) Diagnosis: Diagnosis is primarily clinical. There is evidence of a degree of dementia, hyperreflexia (including preserved ankle jerks), and posterior column signs suggesting spinal cord involvement rather than peripheral neuropathy. MRI scan is negative for other etiologies, such as lymphoma. Patients with transverse myelitis usually have a distinct spinal cord level of sensory/motor involvement. When sensory involvement is prominent, peripheral neuropathy should be considered.

    c) Treatment: If spasticity is severe, neurological consultation should be considered.

      (1) Use baclofen (Lioresal) 5 mg po tid with dosage increased to 10 mg tid if necessary.

        or

      (2) Use dantrolene (Dantrium) 25 mg po bid with dosage increased to 25 mg qid if necessary.

  2. Transverse myelitis

    a) Clinical presentation: In general, transverse myelitis is uncommon in HIV patients but usually related to herpes zoster, CMV, or spinal lymphoma. It can also be caused by TB spinal abscess or be part of acute HIV seroconversion. The syndrome presents as acute or subacute with onset of motor/sensory dysfunction in the lower extremities, usually with back pain at the level of the involved spinal cord. Evidence of distinct demarcation at the involved level is present.

    b) Diagnosis: CAT scan, or preferably MRI scan, should be obtained to rule out a mass lesion (tumor or abscess). If the scan is normal, then CSF examination should be undertaken for evidence of infection or meningeal lymphomatosis.

    c) Treatment: ZDV therapy is begun if not already being used. Treatment for CMV, in consultation with an infectious disease specialist, may also be warranted.

C. Peripheral neuropathy

  1. Distal symmetric polyneuropathy (DSPN)

    a) Clinical presentation: DSPN affects up to one third of HIV patients and is usually associated with symptomatic HIV infection. Onset is usually subacute with either stocking/glove paresthesias or burning dysesthesias of the soles and distal digits. Clinically, there is loss of ankle jerks and decreased vibration in the toes.

  b) Diagnosis: Nerve conduction studies demonstrate defects in both motor and sensory fibers. Drug-induced neuropathy (e.g., INH, alcohol, vincristine) must be eliminated as a possible etiology.

  c) Treatment: Only palliative treatments are available as follows:

  (1) Nonsteroidal anti-inflammatory drugs (NSAIDs) in appropriate dosages

  or

  (2) Amitriptyline (Elavil) 25 to 50 mg po at night

  or

  (3) Carbamazepine (Tegretol) in appropriate dosages

  (4) Capsaisin 0.025% (Zostrix) topically qid with handwashing after use

  (5) Acupuncture may be helpful in alleviating symptoms.

2. Inflammatory neuropathy (mononeuritis multiplex or inflammatory demyelinating neuropathy)

  a) Clinical presentation: This condition most commonly affects asymptomatic, seropositive patients. Onset is either sudden or with slow progression (days to weeks) of patchy motor/sensory deficits. Cranial nerves are occasionally involved. Etiology is unknown, although immune mediation has been implicated.

  b) Treatment: No consistently effective treatment is available. Plasmapheresis has been effective in some patients.

3. Lumbosacral polyradiculopathy

  a) Clinical presentation: Occurrence is usually in symptomatic AIDS patients. Onset is rapid, with progressive weakness and areflexia of the legs, often with patchy sensory loss and sphincter disturbances. The etiology is unknown, although CMV infection has been implicated. Syphilis should be ruled out in all cases.

  b) Diagnosis: CAT or MRI scan of the lower lumbosacral spine is obtained to eliminate mass lesions or disc disease as possible etiologies. CSF examination frequently reveals an inflammatory picture (> 400 white blood cells [WBCs]/mm^3 and 40% polymorphonuclear granulocytes [PMNs]). CMV is frequently recovered from viral culture. A subgroup of patients have a less inflammatory spinal fluid (< 100 WBCs/mm^3, mostly mononuclear). Some of these cases are due to meningeal involvement with lymphoma and have a more indolent course.

  c) Treatment: Some patients have improved with ganciclovir, but in general, patients proceed rapidly to complete paralysis and death within 2 or 3 months.

4. Autonomic neuropathy: This infrequently occurs in HIV disease. Affected patients may have postural hypotension or cardiovascular instability.

5. Toxic axonal neuropathy: Didanosine and zalcitabine (Hivid) are etiologic agents. Clinical features are similar to those of distal sensory polyneuropathy outlined above. Preexistent neuropathy predisposes the patient to this adverse effect. Symptoms generally resolve if medication is discontinued after development of symptoms.

D. Myopathy

1. Nonspecific myopathy

a) Clinical presentation: Occasionally, patients present asymptomatically, although usually there is progressive muscle aching and/or proximal weakness. The etiology is unclear, although ZDV has been implicated as a possible causative factor.

b) Diagnosis: Elevated muscle enzymes (CPK and/or aldolase) are present. Electromyogram is obtained, if needed, to confirm the diagnosis.

c) Treatment: Discontinue ZDV if causation is suspected.

2. Polymyositis-like syndrome: A syndrome similar to polymyositis has been described with HIV disease.

IX. *MYCOBACTERIUM AVIUM* COMPLEX (MAC)

1. Clinical presentation: MAC is frequently cultured from sputum, even when not causing disease. When disseminated, MAC can present with a variety of manifestations, including adenopathy, hepatosplenomegaly, fevers, night sweats, weight loss, diarrhea, or cytopenia.

2. Diagnosis: Organisms should be cultured from specimens other than sputum (e.g., blood, stool, bone marrow).

3. Treatment: Treatment of MAC is difficult, requiring multidrug regimens in consultation with a specialist. Rifabutin, ethambutol, ciprofloxacin, clarithromycin, clofazimine, and amikacin all show activity against MAC, but exact treatment regimens are not yet defined. Isolation of MAC from sputum alone does not require treatment.

4. Prophylaxis: The FDA has approved rifabutin for use with CD4 of less than 200, although MAC doesn't usually occur until CD4 of less than 100. Prescribe rifabutin (Mycobutin) 150 mg 2 capsules po every day. Recently, identified side effects include iritis and pseudojaundice. Significant drug interactions have been identified with decreased efficacy of methadone, dapsone, and several anticonvulsants. Decreased bioavailability of ZDV has been reported but is of uncertain clinical significance. There is a theoretical concern of emergence of bacterial and mycobacterial resistance in those individuals prophylaxed with rifabutin.

NOTE: A blood culture for MAC should be obtained prior to prophylaxis. Treatment can begin prior to final culture results.

X. IDIOPATHIC THROMBOCYTOPENIA PURPURA (ITP)

A. Clinical presentation: Bruising and petechiae are the most common presenting complaints. However, epistaxis, gingival, and rectal bleeding can occur. Patients with HIV can present with isolated thrombocytopenia as their only manifestation of illness.

B. Treatment: Therapy includes ZDV, ZDV + Dapsone, steroids, danazol, and intravenous gammaglobulin; sometimes splenectomy or plasmapheresis is indicated. Pulse decadron may also be useful in managing chronic ITP. Comanagement with infectious disease, HIV, or hematology specialist is recommended.

6

HIV Infection in Women

GYNECOLOGIC MANAGEMENT GUIDELINES

AIDS is the fourth leading cause of death for women in the United States. In some cities, it is the leading cause of death for women of reproductive age. Any sexually active woman in your practice should be evaluated for her risk of HIV. Socioeconomic status and race cannot be used as a basis for determining risk for HIV.

HIV may manifest differently in women than in men. Some of these manifestations require special attention. The care of women with HIV should encompass the standards for gynecologic care, with special attention given to areas of genital tract infections, cervical dysplasia/cancer, and family planning.

Over 90% of pediatric HIV is attributable to women with HIV transmitting the virus during pregnancy or childbirth (vertical transmission). By providing the best HIV counseling and treatment to women, it may also be possible to reduce the risks associated with vertical transmission.

I. INITIAL VISIT: MEDICAL BASELINE

A. If the patient has had a baseline evaluation, review medical records and laboratory test results to obtain information important for gynecologic evaluation and continued care. Review the following:

1. Risk factors for HIV infection (e.g., injection drug use, sexual activity, blood transfusion)

2. Serological markers of immune status (e.g., CD4 count, CD4 percentage)

3. Tuberculosis and anergy status

4. Medical complications (whether or not related to HIV infection)

5. Medications—continue on HIV medications as appropriate

B. If the patient has not had a baseline medical evaluation, do the following:

1. Initiate baseline evaluation for care of HIV-infected patient (see Chapter 5).

2. Make arrangements for appropriate referral to HIV specialty care, as appropriate.

3. Provide information on HIV disease (see Chapter 1).

C. History

1. Menstrual cycle

   a) Frequency

   b) Duration

   c) Pattern, symptoms

   d) Dates of last menstrual flow

2. Gynecologic history

   a) Pap smear date and results and any special evaluation of abnormal Pap smears. HIV-infected patients have a higher incidence of abnormal Pap smears.

   (1) HPV (human papilloma virus) infection: 18%-49%.

   (2) CIN (cervical intraepithelial neoplasia): 17%-50%

   (3) Cervicitis: 44%

   b) STD (sexually transmitted disease) history

   c) History of Candida vaginitis: Recurrent (chronic) Candida vaginitis can be the first manifestation of HIV progression in women.

   (1) Patients may have HIV-related Candida vaginitis if, in the absence of other etiologies (e.g., diabetes, antibiotics), they have either of the following:

       (a) clinically confirmed chronic Candida that requires constant use of antifungal agents

       (b) annual frequency of infection twice that of baseline

(2) HIV-related vaginal candidiasis occurs with normal CD4 count. Oral and esophageal candidiasis occurs when CD4 counts are less than 500.

d) Sexual/contraceptive history

(1) Inquire about sexual behavior.

(2) Inquire about patients' knowledge of sexual partners' HIV status.

(3) Contraception

(a) Ask about method currently used.

(b) Counsel about effective contraceptive methods.

NOTE: Stress use of condoms for HIV prevention, even if patient is using other contraceptives.

e) Family planning

(1) Provide contraceptive counseling as mentioned earlier.

(2) Encourage the patient to undergo preconception consultation before attempting to become pregnant.

(a) The risk of an HIV-infected woman for bearing a child with HIV is estimated to be 20% to 30%. Factors such as maternal plasma viral load may play a role in vertical transmission.

(b) Consider current medications and teratogenic potential.

3. Past obstetric history

a) Determine gravidity/parity

b) Delivery dates (year) and pregnancy outcome

c) Health status of children

(1) HIV status

(2) Congenital infections

(a) Rubella

(b) Toxoplasmosis

(c) Cytomegalovirus (CMV)

(d) Syphilis

4. Past medical history

a) Review all major medical problems and current therapy.

b) Inquire about past infectious illness (e.g., chickenpox, shingles, herpes, tuberculosis or exposure, parasitic infections, fungal infections).

5. Review of systems (ROS)

a) Usual ROS with attention given to complaints that may signal progression of HIV disease.

b) Review of social and dietary habits that may need modification (e.g., smoking, alcohol and substance use, poor nutrition and sleep habits, environmental hazards).

c) Allergies

II. INITIAL VISIT: PHYSICAL EXAM BASELINE

A. Complete general physical exam (with vital signs, weight)

1. Skin: Look for Kaposi's sarcoma (KS) lesions, warts, psoriasis, seborrhea, syphilitic rash and/or lesions, herpetic lesions, molluscum contagiosum. Check general skin and genital and perirectal area.

2. Fundi (may need to dilate using tropicamide, 0.5%, 1-2 gtts each eye): Look for evidence of retinitis.

3. Oropharynx: Look for leukoplakia, thrush, and KS lesions and assess dental hygiene.

4. Lymph nodes: Look for enlarged nodes.

5. Pulmonary: Assess breath sounds, percussive dullness.

6. Cardiac: routine exam

7. Abdomen: Look for enlarged liver and/or spleen, and note absence of spleen.

8. Nervous system: Look for sensory and motor peripheral neuropathy, early dementia.

B. Gynecologic examination

1. Breast examination

2. Lower abdominal palpation

   a) Assess for masses

   b) Assess for tenderness

3. Examination of genitalia

   a) Examine external genitalia for infection or lesions (e.g., herpes, syphilis, Candida, chancroid).

   b) Examine vagina and cervix for unusual discharge or ulcers. Ulcers should be evaluated for infectious or malignant etiology. CMV infection of the cervix can present as an enlarged, friable, and indurated lesion.

   c) Bimanual exam of uterus and adnexa to evaluate for

      (1) Uterine or adnexal enlargement

      (2) Evidence of pelvic inflammatory disease (PID)

III. BASELINE LABORATORY EVALUATION

A. Routine gynecologic exam

1. Complete blood count (CBC)/differential. In patients with physical exam findings of PID, the white blood cell (WBC) count may be greater than 10,000 only 40% of the time.

2. Pregnancy test (if indicated by history and/or exam)

   a) If positive, counsel about pregnancy and options.

   b) If patient plans to continue pregnancy, see Chapter 7 for more information.

3. Urinalysis, culture (if indicated by history)

4. Venereal Disease Research Laboratory (VDRL)

5. Genital tract screen

    a) Culture for gonorrhea, chlamydia, and other infections as indicated by history or exam.

    b) Pap smear and colposcopy: The Pap smear alone may identify a small number of cases of CIN (about 3%) compared with colposcopy (about 41%). There is no standard as to whether cervical dysplasia screening for HIV patients should be different from that for the general population. Due to the potential disparity between cytological screening and colposcopy, both should be obtained as a baseline.

B. Special gynecologic tests: depends on history, age, and physical exam (e.g., mammogram based on family history, maternal age, or breast exam)

C. Baseline HIV evaluation laboratory tests (if not already obtained)

1. CBC/differential

2. CD4 and percentage of CD4 count

3. HBsAg (hepatitis B surface antigen) screen

4. PPD (tuberculin skin test)

    a) Use Mantoux test: 5 tuberculin units intradermal.

    b) Anergy panel: Use two delayed-type hypersensitivity (DTH) antigens (Candida, mumps, tetanus toxoid).

    c) Positive if induration is $\geq$ 5 mm. See "Common Medical Problems Encountered in HIV Disease" in Chapter 5 for more information on evaluation and management.

5. Liver function tests, electrolytes, chest X-ray if indicated

D. Special laboratory tests/evaluation

1. Culture/biopsy or consultation if suspicious lesions or masses are found on general physical exam.

2. If not sure of finding, refer to HIV specialist for appropriate workup.

IV. FOLLOW-UP AND MANAGEMENT

A. Immediate treatment

1. Based on results of physical exam and lab evaluation

2. Refer to appropriate section of Chapter 5 for suggested treatment or referral to specialists.

3. If the patient is to be treated for PID, consider the following:

    a) HIV-infected patients may not have an elevated WBC count.

    b) HIV-infected patients with PID are more likely to develop a tubal/ovarian abscess and require surgical intervention.

    c) Hospitalize patients and give parenteral antibiotics as recommended by Centers for Disease Control (CDC) guidelines.

B. Contraceptive counseling

    1. Contraception in women with HIV may require two approaches—one for maximum pregnancy prevention and one for disease prevention.

    2. Condoms used correctly in conjunction with the spermicidal agent nonoxynol-9 are effective for both pregnancy and disease prevention. However, there is some concern that nonoxynol-9 may cause mucosal irritation and inflammation and perhaps increase the possibility of transmission. Applying nonoxynol-9 to the wrist is a good test for sensitivity.

    3. Another effective approach is to use a combination of hormonal contraception for maximum pregnancy prevention and condoms for prevention of HIV transmission.

    4. Surgical sterilization can be used for standard gynecologic indications. It should not be recommended only because of the patient's HIV status.

C. Referrals—medical/social services/psychological

    1. Community-based HIV support services

    2. Counseling, as needed

    3. Nutrition consultation

    4. HIV specialty care

D. Return visits and evaluation

    1. Routine follow-up interval if no specific problems—every 6 months

    2. History reevaluation: Pay special attention to any changes in menses, STDs, Candida vaginitis.

    3. Physical reexamination

        a) Repeat gynecologic examination

        b) Careful examination for any suspicious skin lesions

    4. Follow-up laboratory/screening evaluation

        a) CBC, CD4 count, and percentage of CD4 count (if not obtained within past month by other medical follow-up)

        b) Repeat genital tract screening

        c) Screening for cervical dysplasia: There are no established guidelines available for follow-up screening of cervical dysplasia in HIV patients. The CDC has suggested yearly screening if the Pap test specimen is adequate for evaluation. However, this is not different from what is done for HIV-negative patients. Until more specific guidelines are available, an alternative approach based on CD4 counts and Pap test results can be used. In reports of HIV-infected patients with cervical dysplasia, most of the patients had CD4 counts that were less than 500 and frequently had evidence of cervicitis.

(1) CD4 count > 500: Follow with repeat Pap screens if
    (a) baseline colposcopy was normal
    (b) no symptoms or physical findings are suspicious
    (c) Pap smear results are adequate for complete interpretation (endocervical cells present, no atypia present).

(2) CD4 count < 500 or abnormal Pap result: Follow with repeat colposcopic examinations.

7

HIV Infection in Pregnant Patients

MANAGEMENT GUIDELINES

Information about HIV infection during pregnancy is limited. Epidemiological data regarding HIV infection in women indicate that the seroprevalence rate is highest among women of childbearing age and that the percentage of women with AIDS has been increasing over the past decade. Currently, about 11% of people with AIDS in the United States are female.

HIV can be vertically transmitted to the fetus. The risk of vertical transmission is between 20% and 30% if the mother is asymptomatic for HIV infection. Data regarding several aspects of HIV infection during pregnancy are still being developed and include the following:

- Whether or not prognostic markers have the same value in pregnant patients as in nonpregnant patients
- Teratogenic risk of pharmacological therapy (prophylactic or therapeutic) during pregnancy
- Benefit of prophylactic therapy in preventing vertical transmission
- Risk of invasive procedures increasing vertical transmission

Existing management guidelines of HIV infection in pregnant patients are based on modifications of established management principles of obstetric care that have been combined with management protocols used with nonpregnant patients. These guidelines are based on the assumption that it is already known that the patient is infected with HIV (symptomatic or asymptomatic). The usual standards of obstetric care should be used for all patients. In-depth counseling about certain risks and, possibly, avoiding certain procedures should be provided. Care of the HIV-infected pregnant patient must be carried out in conjunction with other health care colleagues who are familiar with caring for and addressing the social needs of these patients.

I. PREGNANCY COUNSELING

When a woman with HIV becomes pregnant or when a pregnant patient learns she is HIV infected, she must receive appropriate counseling and education regarding vertical transmission, health care, treatment options, and available support so that she can make informed decisions.

II. ANTEPARTUM CARE

A. Initial visit: Medical baseline
  1. If the patient has undergone baseline evaluation, review medical records and laboratory test results to obtain information that will be important to obstetric care.
     a) Risk factors for HIV infection (e.g., sexual activity, blood transfusion, injection drugs—pregnancy is generally considered grounds for an emergency admission to a methadone program)
     b) Serological markers of immune status (e.g., CD4 count, CD4 percentage)
     c) Tuberculosis and anergy status
     d) Medical complications (whether related to HIV infection or not)
     e) Medications, clinical trial protocols: If the patient is on any form of therapy for HIV, this should be continued after consideration of potential risks and discussion with the patient.
  2. For newly diagnosed pregnant patients
     a) Initiate baseline evaluation for care of HIV-infected patient.
     b) Make arrangements for appropriate referral to other health care providers' support services.
     c) Provide patient with information related to her HIV status.

B. Initial visit: Obstetric baseline (Database: history)

  1. +Current obstetric data relating to menstrual cycle, to help date the pregnancy

  2. Past obstetric history, with emphasis placed on potentially recurrent obstetric/medical problems

    a) Preterm delivery

    b) Pregnancy loss (miscarriage intrauterine demise, neonatal death)

    c) Abruption, placenta previa

    d) Gestational diabetes

    e) Pregnancy-induced hypertension

    f) Fetal/neonatal problems (intrauterine growth retardation, birth defects, chromosomal problems, infant with HIV infection)

  3. Past medical history: Include review of

    a) Hypertensive disorders

    b) Hematologic disorders

    c) Cardiorespiratory disease

    d) Diabetes

    e) Renal disease

    f) Hepatic disease

    g) Neurological disease

    h) Infection history (measles, chickenpox, tuberculosis or recent exposure, herpes, parasitic, fungal)

  4. Review of systems (ROS)

    a) Perform usual ROS with attention to distinguishing between complaints that may be normal for pregnancy from those that could be signals of progression of HIV disease. (See "Common Medical Problems Encountered in HIV Disease" in Chapter 5.)

    b) Review of social and dietary habits that may need modification during pregnancy (e.g., smoking, alcohol and substance use, poor nutrition and sleep habits, environmental hazards)

    c) Allergies

  5. Family history

    a) History of birth defects or chromosomal or metabolic illness that may be transmittable and may require special counseling or prenatal diagnosis

    b) Special screening/testing (e.g., hemoglobinopathies, metabolic defects) appropriate to ethnic background

C. Physical

  1. Complete general physical exam (with vital signs, weight)

    a) Skin: Look for Kaposi's sarcoma (KS) lesions, warts, psoriasis, seborrhea, syphilitic rash/lesions, herpetic lesions, molluscum contagiosum. Check general skin, genital, and perirectal area.

b) Fundi (may need to dilate using tropicamide 0.5% 1-2 gtts each eye): Look for evidence of retinitis.

c) Oropharynx: Look for leukoplakia, thrush, KS lesions; assess dental hygiene.

d) Lymph nodes: Look for enlarged nodes.

e) Pulmonary: Assess breath sounds, percussive dullness.

f) Cardiac: Perform routine exam.

g) Abdomen: Look for enlarged liver and/or spleen; note absence of spleen.

h) Nervous system: Look for sensory and motor peripheral neuropathy, early dementia.

2. Obstetric

a) Assess uterine size (abdominal/pelvic exam)

b) Assess for fetal life (heart tones, if possible)

3. Gynecologic

a) General pelvic exam with emphasis placed on evidence of infectious problems (lesions, discharge)

b) Assess cervix status (closed, dilated, effaced).

c) Assess vaginal status—normal/abnormal discharge. Test for ruptured membranes if indicated.

D. Laboratory evaluation

1. If the patient has had recent baseline medical evaluation for HIV, review the results. Obtain following tests if not already done.

a) Complete blood count

b) CD4 count

c) Blood type, Rh and antigen titer screen

d) Urinalysis and culture

e) Venereal Disease Research Laboratory (VDRL) and rubella immunity status

f) HBsAg (hepatitis B surface antigen) screen

g) Screen for gestational diabetes

h) Genital tract screen

(1) Sexually transmitted diseases: Gonorrhea, chlamydia, and other infections as may be indicated by history or exam.

(2) Pap smear and/or colposcopy for cervical cancer (see gynecologic management under "Physical" in this section)

2. Special testing/investigation

a) Discuss/order maternal serum alpha-fetoprotein (MSAFP), human chorionic gonadotropin (β-HCG), and estradiol to screen for neural tube defects, chromosome abnormalities.

b) Toxoplasmosis and cytomegalovirus antibody screen

    c) PPD (tuberculin skin test)

      (1) Use Mantoux text—5 tuberculin units intradermal.

      (2) Anergy panel: Use one or two delayed-type hypersensitivity (DTH) antigens (Candida, mumps, tetanus toxoid).

      (3) Positive if induration is ≥ 5 mm. (Refer to tuberculosis section under "Common Medical Problems Encountered in HIV Disease" in Chapter 5.)

    d) Ultrasound examination

      (1) Perform as soon as possible if clinical dates are uncertain or clinically indicated (e.g., vaginal bleeding).

      (2) Baseline 16 to 20 weeks for growth and to confirm dating

    e) Prenatal diagnosis—amniocentesis, percutaneous umbilical blood sampling (PUBS), cardiovascular system (CVS): Discuss and perform as indicated. Special testing may be indicated on the basis of past obstetric or family history or as a result of maternal age or test indicating potential fetal risk. At the present time, it is not known if these procedures will increase the risk of perinatal transmission of HIV. These invasive procedures can be associated with bleeding between the fetus and mother. This raises concern about possible inoculation of the fetus with the virus during such procedures. The patient should be extensively counseled about her risks and options. This should be well documented in the patient's chart. If one of these procedures is indicated and necessary for providing care, then it may be appropriate to proceed.

E. Follow-up obstetric/medical care

  1. Reinforce patient's knowledge of HIV as needed during follow-up visits.

  2. Request dietary consultation

  3. Patient can be followed at usual obstetric intervals if the pregnancy is not complicated by medical or obstetric conditions that warrant more frequent visitation.

  4. Symptoms of HIV disease progression can be subtle and could be regarded as complaints not uncommon in pregnancy. Patients should be instructed to call with any complaints that are unusual for them. Attention should be given to

    a) Central nervous system (CNS): headaches, visual disturbance, mental status changes

    b) Respiratory: difficulty breathing, cough (productive, nonproductive)

    c) Gastrointestinal: diarrhea, weight loss, dysphagia/odynophagia

    d) Gynecologic: vaginitis (see gynecologic management under "Physical" in this section): Evaluate or refer for medical evaluation for symptoms or findings (low CD4 percentage/count) that suggest HIV progression (see Chapter 5).

  5. Repeat testing/special evaluation

    a) Ultrasound

   (1) Repeat growth assessment at 28 to 30 weeks.
   (2) Repeat growth assessment every 4 weeks if obstetric/medical factors
       indicate risk for growth abnormality (e.g., hypertensive disease, dia-
       betes, drug use, alcohol use, renal disease, previous intrauterine
       growth retardation [IUGR], collagen vascular disease, multifetal preg-
       nancy).
   (3) Evaluate obstetric complications (e.g., bleeding).
  b) Fetal nonstress test, biophysical profile: Order as indicated by obstet-
     ric/medical condition.
  c) Laboratory evaluation
   (1) Monitor CD4 percentage/count every 3 months.
   (2) Repeat screen for diabetes at 28 to 30 weeks if earlier screening was
       indicated and result was negative.
   (3) Repeat VDRL testing sometime prior to admission for delivery.
   (4) Repeat other laboratory evaluation as indicated by medical problems
       (renal disease, systemic lupus erythematosus [SLE]) or necessary for
       monitoring HIV care.
   (5) Screening for cervical dysplasia: There are no established guidelines
       available for follow-up screening of cervical dysplasia in HIV patients.
       The Centers for Disease Control has suggested yearly evaluation if the
       Pap test specimen is adequate for evaluation. However, this is not
       different from what is done for HIV-negative patients. Until more
       specific guidelines are available, an alternative approach based on CD4
       counts and Pap test results can be used. In reports of HIV-infected
       patients with cervical dysplasia, most of the patients had CD4 counts
       that were less than 500 and frequently had evidence of cervicitis.
       (a) CD4 count of more than 500: Follow with repeat Pap screens if
          (i) Baseline colposcopy is normal.
          (ii) No symptoms or physical findings are suspicious.
          (iii) Pap smear results are adequate for complete interpretation
               (endocervical cells present, no atypia present).
       (b) CD4 count of less than 500 or abnormal Pap result: Follow with
           repeat colposcopic examinations.
F. Medical therapy for HIV infection in pregnancy
   Much concern about potential risks to the fetus surrounds the therapeutic agents
   used in management of HIV infection. Although information about the teratogenic risks of some agents may be known, information is lacking about newer
   agents that are being developed. Accordingly, there can be variation of opinion
   on using these agents. Any policy regarding this is likely to change as more
   information is learned. The most controversial area of medical therapeutics is
   that of prophylaxis. The following is given as a guideline. Whether medical
   therapy is for treatment of symptomatic disease or is prophylactic, individualiza-

tion is necessary. Decisions should be made jointly by the obstetrician, internist, and the patient.

1. Established medical treatment—should be maintained
2. New medical treatment
   a) Therapeutic
      (1) Based on definitive diagnosis of HIV-related condition (see appropriate section in Chapter 5 for illness in question).
      (2) Preserving the health of the woman should be the primary consideration driving decisions to pursue new courses of therapy.
      (3) Increase frequency of follow-up visits as necessary to look for adverse side effects and follow progress of therapy.
   b) Prophylactic
      (1) Discuss the risks and benefits of therapy with the patient.
      (2) Offer the patient the opportunity to start therapy if she so desires.
      (3) Do appropriate follow-up visits for monitoring for side effects.
      (4) Prevention of maternal-fetal transmission: An interim analysis of ACTG 076 demonstrated in pregnant women with CD4 counts over 200 that zidovudine (ZDV) given to the mother antepartum and intrapartum, and also given to the neonate, lowered transmission of HIV to the fetus when compared to controls. General recommendations for the use of ZDV in pregnant women have not been made at the time of this writing because analysis and discussion of this study continue.

III. INTRAPARTUM CARE

The important aspects of intrapartum care center around the potential for nosocomial spread (to neonate or health care workers) of HIV. This risk emanates from the exposure to potentially infectious blood and body fluids normally encountered during the delivery process.

A. Labor and delivery admission procedures
   1. Obtain and review updated prenatal records.
   2. Obtain an interval history and review of systems since last prenatal visit, with emphasis on reason for admission such as
      a) Signs of labor
      b) Rupture of membranes (with or without labor)
      c) Vaginal bleeding
      d) Hypertension
      e) Scheduled admission for induction or cesarean section

3. Physical examination (Follow the guidelines of universal precautions in Appendix 7–A, in this chapter.)

   a) Complete general physical examination. Special attention should be directed toward parts of the examination that could reveal problems as suggested by symptoms revealed in the history.

   b) Document

      (1) Patient's vital signs

      (2) Uterine activity pattern

      (3) Fetal status (heart rate, presentation)

   c) Pelvic examination (digital, speculum, or none) as warranted by the admission history

   d) Genital cultures as indicated by the history and exam (e.g., infectious screening in cases of preterm premature rupture of the membranes, ulcerative lesions suggestive of herpes simplex)

   e) Ultrasound examination as directed by history or physical findings (e.g., clarify fetal presentation, assess for fetal growth retardation and placental location)

4. Laboratory assessment: routine admission laboratory test results. Additional laboratory test results may be indicated by history, examination, or as part of continued antepartum HIV surveillance plan (use universal precautions when obtaining blood or starting IV).

5. Notify pediatrician of patient's admission.

6. Notify anesthesiologist of patient's admission.

B. Continuing intrapartum care

   1. Fetal assessment

      a) Electronic fetal heart rate monitoring: Noninvasive external monitoring is suggested. The patient should be informed of the controversy surrounding this issue—that is, the theoretical concern that fetal scalp electrode monitoring might increase the risk of perinatal transmission of HIV.

      b) Fetal scalp blood sampling should be avoided for the reasons indicated above. If there is a question about the fetal acid base status, then an internal scalp electrode can provide adequate information that could avoid having to perform an operative delivery for presumed fetal distress.

   2. Uterine activity monitoring: external or internal monitoring as indicated by clinical conditions

   3. If amniotic membranes rupture spontaneously or have to be ruptured artificially, then universal precautions regarding contact with body fluids and blood should be observed.

   4. Maternal assessment

      a) Standard assessment of vital signs and progress of labor

      b) Special monitoring and assessment as dictated by obstetric/medical problems, such as

      (1) Abruption

      (2) Hypertensive disorders

      (3) Diabetes

      (4) Cardiac/renal/pulmonary disease

   c) Obtain consultation with other medical specialties as indicated by patient's medical status

5. Analgesia

   a) Intravenous narcotics: These can be used as needed and indicated by clinical condition of patient.

   b) Regional analgesia (e.g., epidural block)

      (1) This should have been discussed during prenatal care visits.

      (2) Inform patient that opinions about use of this type of therapy may vary among anesthesiologists.

      (3) There may be concern about whether or not the procedure might increase risk of introducing HIV into the CNS.

      (4) It can be used if patient and anesthesiologist agree.

C. Delivery

   1. Route of delivery (vaginal or cesarean section) is chosen on the basis of obstetric/medical indications.

   2. Follow universal precautions for vaginal or cesarean birth.

   3. Use double-glove technique.

   4. For suctioning of infant airway, use DeLee suction attached to low-pressure (140 mm Hg) wall suction or use a bulb suction apparatus. Care should be taken not to cause trauma of infant airway structures.

   5. Obtain additional umbilical cord blood for assessment of neonate's baseline HIV status.

   6. Wash blood and body fluids from the infant's body.

IV. POSTPARTUM CARE

The following are important aspects of the postpartum care of the HIV-infected patient:

A. Efforts to prevent nosocomial infection

   1. Follow universal precautions for handling blood and body fluids.

   2. Counsel mother to avoid breast-feeding.

B. Close observation for HIV progression

   1. Infectious complications are not uncommon in patients in the postpartum period. However, data indicate that HIV-infected pregnant patients may be especially prone to more serious infectious complications.

2. Review all admission laboratory results to assess for any indicators of disease progression (e.g., thrombocytopenia, low CD4 counts, if obtained).

3. Do appropriate evaluation of any pulmonary complaints or alterations of mental status.

C. Contraceptive counseling

1. Patients should be counseled on how to avoid unplanned future pregnancies via appropriate contraceptive methods.

2. The type of contraceptive used should be based on effectiveness, patient acceptance of the method, and consideration of the medical status of the patient (see "Follow-Up and Management" in Chapter 6).

   a) Regardless of the contraceptive method, patients should continue to practice safer sex. Condoms should still be used to prevent sexual transmission of HIV.

   b) Oral contraceptives, although effective, should not be used in patients who have hepatic complications of HIV infection or who are on medications that can cause hepatic dysfunction (e.g., dapsone, isoniazid, ketoconazole, sulfamethoxazole-trimethoprin, 5-flucytosine).

   c) Reinforce the importance of the patient's informing her sexual partner(s) as to risk for contracting HIV (see "Assessing Coping Skills" in Chapter 1).

D. Appropriate referrals for follow-up care

1. Pediatric

2. Baseline evaluation in hospital: Continue outpatient follow-up for at least 15 months to determine if HIV infection is evident.

   a) By serological testing

   b) By the development of clinical disease consistent with HIV infection

3. Medical/gynecologic

   a) Continued care by medical/gynecologic team if patient was previously under their care for known HIV infection

   b) Make a new referral if patient is newly diagnosed and has not had a baseline evaluation.

4. Social services

   a) Continued social services support for patient previously being seen by social worker or patient advocate group

   b) New referral for patients who were recently diagnosed and not yet informed of support service support programs

   c) Referral for infant care needs or arrangements for infant care, as appropriate

Appendix 7–A: Universal Precautions

1. Wash your hands *before* and *after* all patient or specimen contact.
2. Handle all human blood and certain body fluids (any body fluid containing visible blood; semen; vaginal secretions; cerebrospinal, pleural, peritoneal, and amniotic fluid) as potentially infectious.
3. Universal precautions do not apply to feces, nasal secretions, sputum, saliva, sweat, tears, urine, or vomitus unless they contain visible blood.
4. Wear personal protective equipment (PPE) for potential contact with blood and body fluids. PPE includes, but is not limited to, gloves, goggles, gowns, or aprons.
5. *Do not recap* or manipulate used needles. Immediately after use, place in a rigid impermeable container.
6. Handle soiled linen as little as possible. Wash separately in hot soapy water. One cup of bleach may be used if appropriate.
7. Spills of blood or body fluids must be handled carefully; gloves must be worn. Spills should be absorbed by paper towels and the area cleaned with 1:10 solution of bleach (1 part bleach to 9 parts water).
8. Soiled dressings should be double bagged and placed in an outside residential trash barrel with a lid.
9. All procedures are performed in a manner that minimizes splash, spray, splatter, and the generation of droplets.

8

Experimental and
Complementary Therapies

Current treatment choices for management of HIV disease are limited. Many investigational therapies are available as treatment options to primary care providers and offer expanded options for disease management. Accessing investigational new drugs (INDs) through IND or parallel track protocols and clinical trials may provide patients with their best hope when other forms of treatment fail.

Much research is also being done on HIV therapy that falls outside the realm of traditionally approved medications. Many nontraditional interventions, such as acupuncture, Chinese herbs, and meditation, have been reported to provide symptom relief. Studies are currently under way to assess their effect on immune function and other bodily functions. Sometimes, additional psychological benefit is derived from patients choosing these therapies as a means of exercising control.

Providers should inquire about and monitor nontraditional treatments used by their patients. Supporting patients pursuing complementary therapies is helpful as long as the therapy is not harming them.

Accessing Experimental Therapies

AIDS CLINICAL TRIALS GROUP (ACTG)

AIDS clinical trials are federally funded studies of INDs, such as antivirals, vaccines, immunomodulators, and prophylaxis, and treatment of opportunistic infections and neoplasms, as well as other approaches to controlling the virus itself. See the resource section at the end of this chapter for information on how to find the ACTG.

COMMUNITY-BASED CLINICAL TRIALS

Community-based clinical trials may be sponsored by the government, foundations, or private drug companies. Patients can participate through their primary care providers, without having to visit additional research sites. There is a national network of community research initiatives that coordinates community-based clinical trials. If your community has a large HIV-positive patient population, you can contact one of these organizations about enrolling your patients in their studies. See the resource section at the end of this chapter for information on how to find the community research initiative nearest you.

COMPASSIONATE USE

Sometimes pharmaceutical companies will make a promising drug available prior to its approval on a compassionate use basis. Usually, to obtain these drugs for your patient, you must be able to document that existing therapy is ineffective. Even after approval, some companies make drugs available for free when a patient can't pay. For details, contact the manufacturer of the particular drug desired.

PARALLEL TRACK (EXPANDED ACCESS)

Parallel track is an FDA program that expands access to a promising drug that has not yet been approved. This is for individuals who do not meet the entry criteria, who do not have access to clinical trials in progress, or who have failed on approved therapies. Drugs offered under this program show sufficient efficacy to warrant wider release. Contact the manufacturer to receive an application for investigator status within the parallel track system.

Complementary Therapies

ACUPUNCTURE

Many patients report acupuncture as being effective in alleviating symptoms, especially neuropathy, gastrointestinal disorders, cravings, anxiety, and fatigue. Some providers are having success using acupuncture for detoxification and treating addiction. Studies documenting the effects of acupuncture are ongoing at this time.

HERBS

Evidence suggests that many herbs possess pharmacological properties. Some studies are under way to assess the effects of specific herbal remedies on HIV disease. Because these substances are not under FDA control, your patients may be self-medicating. Some of these substances can have a profound effect on internal organs and systems and may interact with medications. It is important for you to be aware of any herbal or nutritional remedies your patients are taking. Encourage patients seeking herbal therapies to consult with a trained acupuncturist, herbalist, or naturopath.

CHIROPRACTIC THERAPY

Chiropractic therapy is the attempt to restore normal function of the nervous system by manipulating and treating the structures of the human body, especially the spinal column. Many patients report symptom relief associated with aches and pains, lack of joint mobility, and stress and tension as a result of chiropractic care.

MASSAGE

Massage has been documented to improve circulation and lymphatic function, increase energy, provide relaxation, and create a feeling of wellness. Also, it feels good. The therapeutic benefits of touch cannot be underestimated.

MEDITATION

This practice provides a form of mental relaxation and reduces the effects of stress.

VITAMINS

Vitamin deficiency is common in HIV patients. Supplementary vitamin therapy may be helpful.

EXERCISE

Exercise has been shown to improve immune function, reduce stress, and counteract insomnia.

DIET

Nutrition plays a very important role in a person's overall health and healing. Consultation with a nutritionist may be helpful.

EMPOWERMENT PROGRAMS

Many programs such as workshops, healing circles, support groups, and retreats that promote acceptance of self and taking control of one's life have been used by people with HIV to improve the quality of their lives.

Resources

RESOURCES FOR CLINICAL TRIALS INFORMATION

Project Inform
347 Dolores, Suite 301
San Francisco, CA 94110 1-800-822-7422

Drug Trials Information Hot Line
National Institutes of Health . . . . 1-800-TRIALS A

This resource has a comprehensive listing of all HIV-related clinical trials in the United States, including entry criteria and how to enroll.

Experimental Treatment Hotline
In New York City: 1-800-633-7444
Outside New York City: . . . . (212) 239-5523

NEWSLETTERS

AmFAR Experimental Treatment Directory
1515 Broadway
New York, NY 10036 . . . . (212) 719-0033

Treatment Issues
GMHC Dept. of Medical Information
129 W 20th Street
New York, NY 10023 . . . . (212) 807-6655

AIDS Treatment News
PO Box 411256
San Francisco, CA 94141 . . . . (415) 255-0588

BETA
SF AIDS Foundation
PO Box 6182
San Francisco, CA 94101 . . . . (415) 863-AIDS

9

Guidelines for HIV-Infected Children and Adolescents or Those Suspected of Being HIV Infected

HIV infection in children and adolescents poses special challenges. Typically, young children acquire HIV prenatally or perinatally. Adolescents more typically acquire HIV through their own high-risk behavior. All adolescents should be routinely evaluated for risk and counseled appropriately. Infants and young children born to mothers who have HIV or who are at risk should also be evaluated.

HIV often presents differently in children than in adults. These guidelines assist the practitioner with effective diagnosis and management.

Emotional support and social service referral are especially important to the child and his or her family.

I. PRIMARY WELL-CHILD CARE AND FOLLOW-UP

A. Document history, mode of transmission

NOTE: See Appendixes 9–A and 9–B in this chapter for sample letters to facilitate communication between the primary care provider and the infectious disease specialist.

B. Schedule of primary care visits

1. Prenatal: counseling and referral to pediatric HIV specialist

2. Newborn: perinatal visit with counseling, referral to pediatric HIV specialist if not made earlier—hepatitis B virus (HBV)

3. 2 weeks: first well-child visit

4. 2 months: well-child visit—diphtheria, pertussis, and tetanus (DPT); inactive polio vaccine (IPV); HiBCV; HBV

5. 4 months: well-child visit—DPT, IPV, HiBCV

6. 6 months: well-child visit—DPT, IPV, HiBCV (optional)

7. 9 months: well-child visit—HBV

8. 12 months: well-child visit

9. 15 months: well-child visit—measles, mumps, rubella (MMR); HiBCV

10. 18 months: well-child visit—DPT, IPV

11. 24 months: well-child visit—pneumovax

12. Over 24 months: individualized care based on particular needs and status of patient

NOTE: Regular oral polio vaccine immunizations should be changed to IPV for infants at risk. Influenza vaccine should be given each year prior to flu season after 6 months of age—in the first year of life, 2 doses, 1 month apart; 1 dose per year thereafter.

C. Points to remember regarding children with HIV

1. Common infections and serious bacterial infections of the lungs and blood are typical; opportunistic infections are *not* the norm.

2. Frequent fever (several times/week or even daily) without obvious underlying cause is sometimes observed.

3. Multiple infections may coexist.

D. Common presenting problems

1. Fever

   a) Possible causes—sepsis/bacteremia, pneumonia, otitis media, and other infections

   b) Fever, no additional symptoms

      (1) Evaluation: Do history and physical, complete blood count (CBC) with differential, blood culture. If culture is abnormal, consider chest X-ray (CXR), pulse oximetry, urinalysis (UA), urine culture, lumbar puncture (LP).

      (2) Intervention: Hospitalize *if* doubts exist about accessibility to follow-up or home care. May treat with oral antibiotics with 24- to 48-hour follow-up.

   c) Recurrent fever, no additional symptoms

      (1) Evaluation: Consider CBC with differential, blood culture.

(2) Intervention: May follow closely without medication.

d) Fever with additional symptoms

(1) Evaluation: Do full sepsis workup, including CBC with differential, blood culture, LP, urine C&S, UA, CXR, pulse oximetry.

(2) Intervention: Contact pediatric infectious disease specialist; implement broad-spectrum antibiotic coverage.

2. Diarrhea and vomiting

a) Possible causes

(1) Bacterial: Salmonella, Shigella, Campylobacter, *Escherichia coli, Clostridium difficile, Aeromonas hydrophilia.*

(2) Viral: Rotavirus, Norwalk agent, enteric adenovirus

(3) Mycobacterial: *Mycobacterium avium*

(4) Protozoal: Cryptosporidium

b) Acute diarrhea, initially without vomiting

(1) Evaluation: Do stool guaiac, stool C&S/O&P, white blood cell (WBC) smear, rotazyme. If positive for Salmonella or Campylobacter, get a blood culture.

(2) Intervention: Implement hydration, specific antibacterial treatment as indicated; treat all Salmonella infections; contact pediatric infectious disease specialist.

c) Chronic diarrhea, with/without weight loss, fever, sweats, and cachexia

(1) Evaluation: as above, additional stool for Mycobacterium

(2) Intervention: calorie supplement

3. Pulmonary

a) Possible causes

(1) Bacterial: *Hemophilus influenzae* Type B (HIB), Mycoplasma, *Streptococcus pyogenes* (gp A), *Staphylococcus aureus, Streptococcus pneumoniae*

(2) Viral: respiratory syncytial virus (RSV), rhinovirus, adenovirus, parainfluenza, influenza, varicella, measles, cytomegalovirus (CMV)

(3) Opportunistic: *Pneumocystis carinii* pneumonia (PCP), CMV, Legionella, Mycobacterium, fungi, parasites

(4) Other: lymphocytic interstitial pneumonia (LIP) or pulmonary lymphohyperplasia, pulmonary manifestations or other organ system disease

NOTE: Two or more of the above may coexist.

b) Acute respiratory decompensation

(1) Evaluation: Perform history and physical, including PPD (tuberculin skin test) status, CBC with differential, CXR, pulse oximetry or arterial blood gases (ABGs), blood culture; obtain specimen for urine testing

if necessary; obtain sputum samples; perform bronchoscopy and lung aspiration.

  (2) Intervention: If lobar infiltrate and increased WBC, presumptively treat with broad-spectrum antibiotics; do ABGs follow-up within 48 hours. Consider hospitalization if severely ill; contact pediatric infectious diseases specialist if diagnostic dilemma exists and for specific antiviral therapy.

c) Chronic cough, short of breath (SOB)

  (1) Evaluation: as above, plus PPD with antigenic controls

  (2) Intervention: Consult with infectious disease specialist for comanagement.

4. Candidiasis

a) Presentation: oral candidiasis (thrush), recalcitrant monilial diaper rash, Candida infections of the intertriginous areas (axilla, neck folds, and proximal neck folds)

NOTE: If thrush presents with dysphagia, consider Candida esophagitis.

b) Treatment: Thrush should initially be treated with oral nystatin (100,000 U/ml) 2-5 ml by mouth (po) twice a day (bid). If no response, prescribe clotrimazole troche 10 mg po bid. Young infants may take troche inserted into plastic nipple and used as a pacifier. Fluconazole (3-6 mg/kg body weight per dose po, every day [qd]) should be reserved for those cases that do not respond to clotrimazole.

  If a child with thrush develops dysphagia, the possibility of Candida esophagitis should be considered. Suspected Candida esophagitis can be treated with a course of oral ketaconazole, but if a patient's dysphagia does not resolve, endoscopy should be performed. If Candida is confirmed by endoscopy, then the patient should be treated initially with intravenous amphotericin B and later with fluconazole. Cutaneous candidiasis can be treated with topical nystatin or with an imidazole cream.

5. Varicella

a) Exposure: HIV-infected children are at risk for severe and sometimes fatal varicella infections. They should be given VZIG, preferably within 48 hours of a significant exposure to varicella or zoster (shingles), and definitely within 96 hours of the exposure. A significant exposure to varicella or zoster would be

  (1) a continuous household contact

  (2) more than 1 hour of indoor play with a playmate

  (3) direct in-hospital contact.

b) Treatment: Exposure-recommended dose of varicella-zoster immune globulin (VZIG) is 125 units (1 vial) per 10 kg body weight with a maximum dose of 625 units (5 vials). If an HIV-infected child presents with varicella, he or she should be treated with intravenous acyclovir 500 mg/m^2 per dose every 8 hours.

II. RECOMMENDED WORKUP SCHEDULE FOR CHILDREN BORN TO WOMEN WITH HIV

A. Prenatal: counseling and advice regarding risk of transmission

B. Newborn: umbilical cord blood HIV culture, counseling

C. 2 weeks: HIV culture (two within the first 6 months), p24 antigen, CD4 and CD8 counts (PPD on parents)

D. 1 month: HIV culture (two within the first 6 months), HIV serology, p24 antigen, CD4 and CD8 counts, CBC, CMV and HBV serology

E. 3 months: HIV culture (two within the first 6 months), p24 antigen, CD4 and CD8 counts, CBC, immunoglobulins (Igs)

F. 6 months: HIV, enzyme-linked immunosorbent assay (ELISA) and Western blot (WB), HIV culture, p24 antigen, CD4 and CD8 counts, liver function tests (LFTs), PPD, Ig levels, and developmental evaluation

G. 9 months: CD4 and CD8 counts, CBC, Igs (repeat optional)

H. 12 months: HIV, ELISA and WB, HIV culture, p24 antigen, CD4 and CD8 counts, LFTs, oximetry, developmental evaluation

I. 15 months: HIV, ELISA and WB, p24 antigen, CD4 and CD8 counts, CBC

J. 18 months: HIV, ELISA and WB, p24 antigen, CD4 and CD8 counts, CBC, Igs (optional), depending on prior results and developmental evaluation

K. Over 24 months: individualized care based on particular needs and status of patient

- Although all of these tests are available to pediatricians (with exception of HIV culture), it may be advisable to comanage these babies with a pediatric HIV specialist for this evaluation.

- HIV serology (ELISA and WB). Reversion to seronegative status by 15 months in healthy babies usually is indicative of noninfection. In rare cases, HIV-infected babies fail to make antibodies, but these babies are symptomatic by 15 months.

- If the HIV culture is positive, consider the baby infected. See Appendix 9–C for classification of HIV infection in children.

- Significant elevation in serum IgG in an at-risk infant is highly suggestive of HIV infection. This may be the most sensitive surrogate marker of HIV infection in infants.

III. TREATMENT MODALITIES

NOTE: See Appendix 9–D for child dosage information.

A. Antiretroviral therapies
   1. Zidovudine (ZDV): Use in children less than 3 months old with the following:
      a) Symptomatic HIV infection (CDC classification P2)
      b) Asymptomatic HIV infection with low CD4 count: less than 20% of total T-cells
      c) Dose and formulation: 180 mg/m^2 per dose given every 6 hours; 10 mg/ml
   2. Didanosine and zalcitabine: dosage and formulation—100 mg/m^2 bid; 10 mg/ml
   3. Nevirapine: available only on study protocols
B. *Pneumocystis carinii* pneumonia prophylaxis
   1. Trimethoprim/sulfamethoxazole (TMP/SMX): First choice for most children and infants: dosage—75 mg/m^2 of TMP per dose bid, 3 times/week (Mon., Tues., Wed.) (or 5 mg/kg/day of TMP in 2 divided doses); 375 mg/m^2 of SMX per dose bid, 3 times/week (Mon., Tues., Wed.).
   2. Aerosolized pentamidine: Only for children who are at least 5 years old and cooperative. Some patients may require more frequent treatment (e.g., every 3 weeks): dosage—300 mg in 6 ml of sterile water, inhaled monthly.
   3. Intravenous pentamidine: dosage—4 mg/kg every 2 to 4 weeks
   4. Dapsone: Dosage—1 mg/kg po, qd (100 mg/day maximum dose). The 5 mg/ml formula must be prepared monthly by pharmacist.
C. Treatment for *Pneumocystis carinii* pneumonia
   1. TMP/SMX: 20 mg/kg of TMP per day in four divided doses for infants and children over 2 months of age. Full dose for full course of treatment. The TMP/SMX calculation is generally made on TMP with a fivefold increase on SMX.
      or
   2. Pentamidine IV: These treatments may be combined with steroids.

NOTE: Both treatments should be combined with steroids.

D. Adjunctive treatment
   Intravenous immune globulin (IVIG) is no longer indicated unless more than one episode of serious bacterial infection occurs.

IV. RECOMMENDATIONS FOR DEVELOPMENTAL SERVICES

A. Children born to HIV-positive mothers whose HIV status is indeterminate should have their developmental status monitored in the same manner as children who are not exposed to HIV.
B. Once a child is definitely diagnosed with HIV infection, a developmental evaluation should be performed every 6 months.

C. Children with HIV infection are eligible in some states for early education/special education services even if they do not yet demonstrate a significant delay in two areas of development.

V. SCHOOL

Assist the parent(s) in making decisions regarding disclosure of the child's HIV status to the school. If HIV status is to be disclosed, a primary school official (e.g., school nurse, social worker) will need to be identified. The person(s) receiving information on the HIV status of the child/student must maintain a full working knowledge of current state laws concerning confidentiality and disclosure.

Assist the parent(s) in determining what additional information may be helpful for the primary school official to be made aware of. The following list includes suggested areas of helpful information:

A. Student's HIV status

B. T-cell count/immune status

C. Medications

   1. Side effects that might be observed

   2. Administered by school nurse

D. Observations

   1. Neurological manifestations: developmental, cognitive

   2. Symptoms of infections: fever, respiratory problems, swollen glands, diarrhea

   3. Absenteeism

E. If a child becomes ill at school, the parent and/or guardian should be contacted. If a parent is unavailable and symptoms of infection occur during school, the primary care physician should be notified.

F. Any treatments necessary while in school

G. It is important that school staff inform parent or physician of any possible exposure to chickenpox. Parents/guardians are encouraged to bring their children to their health care provider for VZIG after chickenpox (for further information see Varicella in "Common Presenting Problems" in this chapter).

VI. MEDICAL EVALUATION (AGES 13-18)

A. First visit

   1. Complete medical history

   2. Complete physical examination, including neurological and neuropsychological assessments. Full gynecologic examination for sexually active female adolescents, for those experiencing unexplained gynecologic problems, or if requested.

   3. Diagnostic testing: HIV serology testing with ELISA and WB

B. Second visit
  1. Discussion of diagnosis and various physical manifestations of HIV infection
  2. Discussion of therapeutic interventions (medical and psychosocial)
  3. Continued discussion of medical history

VII. THERAPEUTIC CONSIDERATIONS

A. Medical
  1. Current range of treatments for HIV-related infections and illnesses
  2. Indications for medication, current available medications, doses, routes, and side effects
  3. Need to make treatment decisions in conjunction with relevant adolescent subspecialists
  4. Indications for hospitalization
  5. Availability of clinical trials
  6. Referral to pediatric HIV specialist
B. Psychosocial and educational
  1. Individual and/or family counseling
  2. HIV support group or group therapy
  3. Identification of supportive adult when diagnosis is not disclosed to parent(s)
  4. Referrals to welfare agency and/or financial counseling for Medicaid and other benefits
  5. Referral to other appropriate community agencies who help the HIV-infected individual
  6. Education regarding safer sex practices and notification of sexual partners
  7. Nutritional counseling

History for Adolescents With HIV:
Checklist 1

_____ 1. Reason for referral; source

_____ 2. Explanation of confidentiality

_____ 3. History of sources of medical care and relevant medical history, including major illnesses, medications, hospitalizations, allergies, and immunizations

_____ 4. Substance use or abuse history, including alcohol, tobacco, marijuana, cocaine and crack, opiates, steroids, and other drugs (type, route, injection history, amount, frequency)

_____ 5. Review of systems, including menstrual history

_____ 6. Sexual history

     _____ a) Patterns of sexual relationships, number and sex of sexual partners, age at initiation of sexual intercourse

     _____ b) Types of sexual experiences, specifying oral, vaginal, and anal intercourse

     _____ c) Sexual orientation

     _____ d) Contraception history and current practices, specifying frequency of condom use

     _____ e) Pregnancy history

     _____ f) Sexual abuse

     _____ g) Sexually transmitted diseases

     _____ h) Use of contraceptive (e.g., spermicide, condom) and in what settings

_____ 7. Family history (medical and psychological)

_____ 8. Dietary history

_____ 9. Social history

     _____ a) Living situation

     _____ b) Sources of emotional and social support

     _____ c) Peer relationships

     _____ d) Mental health status

          _____ (1) general mood

          _____ (2) depression

          _____ (3) suicidal ideation/attempts

     _____ e) Education/occupation

     _____ f) Employment status

     _____ g) Legal status (e.g., emancipated)

     _____ h) Legal problems

Specific Elements of Laboratory
Assessment in Adolescents With HIV:
Checklist 2

1. Serum/blood

_____ a) White blood cell count with differential count

_____ b) Platelet count

_____ c) Hemoglobin/hematocrit

_____ d) Liver function tests, creatinine, blood urea nitrogen, total protein/ albumin

_____ e) Rubella titer

_____ f) Screening test for syphilis

_____ g) Sickle cell preparation

_____ h) Toxoplasmosis titers

_____ i) Quantitative immunoglobulins

2. If symptoms warrant

_____ a) Epstein-Barr virus serology

_____ b) Serum cryptococcal antigen titer

_____ c) Blood culture

3. Immunologic assessment

_____ a) HIV antibody test (if indicated and patient consents to testing)

_____ b) CD4, total number and percentage, total lymphocyte count, and CD4/CD8 ratio—initially and every 6 months; if CD4 count approaches 500/mm^3, CD4 and CD8 monitoring should be done every 3 months.

4. Other laboratory tests

_____ a) Urinalysis

_____ b) Urine culture as needed

_____ c) Skin test for tuberculosis (intradermal)

_____ d) Anergy screen (eight items) at the same time as PPD

_____ e) Chest radiography

5. Sexually active teens

_____ a) Pap smear

_____ b) Culture for gonorrhea

_____ c) Culture for chlamydia

_____ d) Wet prep for trichomonads, white blood cells, hyphae

_____ e) Pregnancy test as indicated

Appendix 9–A:
Sample Letter Form to Facilitate Communication
Between Primary Pediatric Provider
and Infectious Disease Specialist

Primary care provider's address

Date _____

Dear _____

_____ was seen at _____

for: _____ scheduled well-child care/physical exam

_____ scheduled follow-up for _____

_____ walk in/acute care.

Significant physical findings/problems:

The following lab tests/X-rays were obtained:

Test	Results	Test	Results

Current medications:

Immunizations given today:

Plan and follow-up:

Please feel free to contact me at _____ with any questions or concerns.

Sincerely,

Primary care provider

Appendix 9–B:
Sample Letter Form to Facilitate Communication
Between the Infectious Disease Specialist
and Primary Pediatric Provider

Infectious disease specialist address

Date _____

Dear _____

_____ was seen in the HIV clinic on _____

at _____

Progress Summary:

Medications: _____

Referrals: _____

Visiting nurse association/Home care: _____

Developmental evaluation: _____

Case management: _____

Please call us with any questions or concerns and keep us informed about any
changes in primary care or any illnesses or infections. Telephone number _____

Sincerely yours,

Infectious disease specialist

Appendix 9–C:
Summary of CDC Classification of
HIV Infection in Children Under 13 Years of Age

Class P0	Indeterminate infection
Class P1	Asymptomatic infection
Subclass A	Normal immune function
Subclass B	Abnormal immune function
Subclass C	Immune function not tested
Class P2	Symptomatic infection
Subclass A	Nonspecific findings
Subclass B	Progressive neurological disease
Subclass C	Lymphoid interstitial pneumonia
Subclass D	Secondary infectious diseases
Category D1	Specified secondary infectious diseases listed in the CDC surveillance definition for AIDS
Category D2	Recurrent serious bacterial infections (e.g., sepsis)
Category D3	Other specified secondary infectious diseases
Subclass E	Secondary cancers
Category E1	Specified secondary cancers listed in the CDC surveillance definition for AIDS
Category E2	Other cancers possibly secondary to HIV infections
Subclass F	Other diseases possibly due to HIV infection

Appendix 9–D:
Pediatric Doses and Formulation

Medication	Formulation	
	Dose	Preparation Strength
TMP/SMX	2.5 mg/kg of TMP per dose bid	40 mg TMP/5 ml
	3 times/week (Mon., Tues., Wed.)	200 mg SMX/5 ml
Dapsone	1 mg/kg qd (100 mg/day maximum dose)	5 mg/ml
IV pentamidine	4 mg/kg q 2-4 weeks	
Aerosolized pentamidine	300 mg in 6 mls of sterile water—inhaled treatment, monthly (for children at least 5 years old who are able to cooperate)	
IVIG	400 mg/kg per dose every month, administered in 4-6 hours	
ZDV	180 mg/m^2 per dose given every 6 hours	10 mg/ml
Didanosine	100 mg/m^2 per dose given bid	10 mg/ml

10

Neuropsychological
Manifestations of HIV Disease

Patients with HIV can present with delirium, an acute confusional state. This is often reversible and must be ruled out as part of the workup for mental status changes. AIDS dementia complex (ADC) and depression are the two most common neuropsychological manifestations of HIV. Development of ADC can be insidious, with symptoms developing gradually over a period of months. Evaluations for ADC may need to be done at several intervals. Depression presents with many similar symptoms and can coexist with ADC. These distinctions are important to make because they have treatment implications.

Assessing for ADC is not unlike assessing for dementia with other etiologies. The degree to which ADC is a complicating factor is different with every individual who is HIV infected. It may occur as one of the early signs of the progression to AIDS with continuing deterioration of certain cognitive functions, or it may arise in the end stage of AIDS. Others may reach the end stage with little or no significant impairment in cognitive functioning. There is evidence that zidovudine (ZDV) helps some patients maintain cognitive functioning.

Ideally, every person who is infected with HIV should receive a thorough neuropsychological examination as soon as possible to establish a baseline of cognitive functioning. This is extremely useful because it serves as a reference point from which to compare future examinations of cognitive functioning that can be used to document any progressive deterioration and also improvement from medication. Patients whose scores on neuropsychological tests indicate cognitive impairment or depression should be referred to psychologists, psychiatrists, or neurologists as appropriate for further workup and treatment.

Unfortunately, neuropsychological examinations are seen as expensive, because they cost about $1,000 to $1,500. However, when compared to the cost of a computerized axial tomography (CAT) scan or magnetic resonance imaging (MRI), they do not seem as expensive, particularly given the utility of the information that can be gathered from a complete neuropsychological workup. There is great interest in a shorter, less expensive neuropsychological screening method that identifies possible deterioration in cognitive functions in those persons who are HIV positive. Presented in this chapter are some screening measures that can help identify persons that might be in need of further assessment for cognitive impairment and/or ADC. It must be emphasized that these are screening measures and impaired performance on these measures does not necessarily indicate the presence of dementia but should trigger a more in-depth neuropsychological and neurological examination.

I. DELIRIUM

A. Presentation: Clinical features develop over a short period of time and tend to fluctuate during the course of the day—characterized by disorganized thinking, decreased level of consciousness, perceptual disturbances, disorientation, memory impairment, change in psychomotor activity, and decreased attention to external stimuli.

B. Cause: Generally, delirium results from opportunistic infections, neoplasms, metabolic disturbances, hematologic problems, or medication. The hypoxia that occurs from these conditions may be just enough to affect brain function and lead to an acute delirium. Additional risk factors include prior brain damage and alcohol or drug addiction.

C. Assessment: A thorough history, along with diagnostic testing for medical conditions that can cause acute mental status changes, must be considered.

II. AIDS DEMENTIA COMPLEX (ADC)

A. Presentation: ADC can appear at any time during illness. Nearly all presentations of ADC are subcortical in nature. Cognitive and motor slowing, tremor or other movement disorders, and apathy are characteristic. Sometimes, in severely ill

TABLE 10.1 Manifestations of ADC

Cognitive	Motor	Behavior	Other
	Early		
Forgetfulness	Slowing	Apathy	Headache
Decreased concentration	Unsteady gait	Social withdrawal	Seizures
Conceptual confusion	Weakness	Agitation	Depression
Information-processing difficulties	Handwriting changes	Altered personality	Psychotic features
Visuospatial disorganization	Hyperreflexia		
	Tremor		
	Clumsiness		
	Speech difficulties		
	Late		
Confusion	Psychomotor retardation	Indifference	Organic psychosis
Memory loss	Ataxia	Wide-eyed stare	Tremor
Global dysfunction	Spasticity	Incontinence	Frontal lobe disturbance
	Weakness	Mutism	
	Dyskinesia		
	Aphasia		
	Parkinsonism		

patients a cortical dementia, characterized by aggression, agitation, apraxia, aphasia, psychosis, memory loss, and global dysfunction, will develop (see Table 10.1).

B. Cause: ADC is caused by toxic effects of HIV in the brain.

C. Assessment: Diagnostic tests that rule out opportunistic infections and neoplasms, which may have symptoms similar to those of ADC, should be done (see "Common Medical Problems Encountered in HIV Disease" in Chapter 5). Assessment of symptom development over time is key in diagnosing ADC. Specific tests that determine whether someone is experiencing subcortical or cortical difficulty exist. Despite the use of diagnostic tools, it may be nearly impossible to distinguish these dementias from each other, and treatments appropriate for both may need to be administered simultaneously. Self-report and reports of significant others about subtle mental status and behavioral changes may be the most important clues in identifying ADC.

III. NEUROPSYCHOLOGICAL TESTING

A. Trail-Making Test

This test is a useful initial screen for cognitive impairment.

The Trail-Making Test is a very quick measure that is sensitive to brain impairment. On Trails A, the subject is asked to connect with a pencil line in numerical order 25 concentric circles without lifting the pencil from the paper. It is important that the subject be given the practice example first and then asked to perform the task as fast as possible. The paper should be anchored in place or held down by the examiner so the subject does not have to contend with paper movement.

Trails B is more difficult and requires the subject to connect concentric circles in sequential order, alternating between circles numbered from 1 to 13 and circles lettered from A to L. Again, it is important to instruct patients to complete this task as fast as they can and to keep the pencil on the paper.

Trails A and B are useful tests because to complete them an integration of several cognitive functions is required, including visual, motor, perceptual, and memory functions. It is important to administer both Trails A and B and to begin with Trails A. This is the standard procedure on which the norms were developed. It is also not uncommon to see good performance on Trails A followed by significantly impaired performance on Trails B. This should not be thought of as a test of primarily subcortical dementia, because lesions in many different areas of the brain can result in impaired performance, many of which can be in cortical areas. Trails A and B generally take less than 5 minutes to administer. The test is available from Reitan Neuropsychology Laboratory, 2920 South 4th Avenue, Tucson, AZ 85713-4819; (602) 882-2022.

Patients with cognitive impairment have a difficult time performing this test, displaying tremendous slowness in their capabilities, getting lost, forgetting the task, taking indirect paths between circles, repeating themselves, or failing to make easy shifts from one set to another.

The value of this test lies in assessing a patient's slowness relative to how others perform. The usefulness of this test increases with the provider's experience in administering it. To achieve a basis of comparison, it is helpful to give the test to individuals who don't have dementia.

B. Other tests for cognitive impairment

1. The Symbol Digit Modalities Test

The Symbol Digit Modalities Test (SDMT) is another quick (5 minutes to administer) test that can easily be added to a screening examination for cognitive impairment. Subjects can give written or spoken responses, so it is not dependent on reading level. The test is relatively free of cultural bias and can be used with people who do not speak English. This test is also a good measure of deterioration over time. This instrument is available from Western Psychological Services, 12031 Wilshire Blvd., Los Angeles, CA 90025-1251; 1-800-648-8857; fax (310) 478-7838.

2. Stroop Neuropsychological Screening Test

Another instrument that has proved a valuable screening for brain impairment is the Stroop Neuropsychological Screening Test (SNST). It takes approximately 5 minutes to administer and claims to differentiate adult brain impairment from nonimpairment in 79% to 92% of cases. This instrument can be ordered from Psychological Assessment Resources, P.O. Box 998, Odessa, FL 33556; 1-800-331-8378; fax 1-800-727-9329.

3. Dementia Rating Scale

Any one or more of the above measures can be used as a screening for cognitive deficits. To obtain a more thorough screen, the Dementia Rating Scale (DRS) can also be added, which takes approximately 15 to 45 minutes to administer. The DRS is made up of questions and tasks that assess attention, initiation/perseveration, construction, conceptualization, and memory. Although it was normed on a sample of healthy adults ranging from 65 to 71 years of age, impaired performance on this measure for adults younger than the normative sample becomes even more significant. It can be very useful to document progression of cognitive decline in the absence of a complete neuropsychological workup. This instrument can be ordered from Psychological Assessment Resources, P.O. Box 998, Odessa, FL 33556; 1-800-331-8378; fax 1-800-727-9329.

4. MicroCog: Assessment of Cognitive Functioning

For those who have computer capabilities and can spend $15.00 per screening exam, MicroCog: Assessment of Cognitive Functioning is an excellent instrument that is computer administered and scored, saving clinician time. You will need to purchase the PsyTest software and the test from The Psychological Corporation, 555 Academic Court, San Antonio, TX, 78204-2498; 1-800-228-0752.

NOTE: All of the above measures can be administered by individuals with limited training. However, the interpretation of the results requires professional training in neuropsychology, psychiatry, or neurology.

IV. FOLSTEIN MINI MENTAL STATUS EXAM[1]

The Folstein Mini Mental Status Exam is one evaluation tool for cognitive impairment. It is not considered part of a standard neuropsychological screening. The care provider does not need to be a psychiatrist to use the Folstein. It is recommended that individuals with total scores of less than 20 points be referred to a psychiatrist.

---

1. Reprinted here with permission from *Journal of Psychiatric Research*, Vol. 12, Folstein/Folstein/McHugh, "The Mini Mental State Exam," 1975, Elsevier Science Ltd., Pergamon Imprint, Oxford, England.

Folstein Mini Mental Status Exam

			Points
1. What is the:	year	_____	(1)
	season	_____	(1)
	date	_____	(1)
	month	_____	(1)
2. Where are we:	state	_____	(1)
	county	_____	(1)
	town	_____	(1)
	hospital	_____	(1)
	floor	_____	(1)
3. Name three objects		_____	(3)
4. Serial 7's [counting by 7s] (5 answers) or spell "world" backwards		_____	(5)
5. Recall three objects		_____	(3)
6. Name a pencil, a watch		_____	(2)
7. Repeat "no ifs, ands, or buts"		_____	(1)
8. Follow 3-step command: Take a paper in your right hand, fold it in half, and put it on the floor		_____	(3)
9. Write a sentence		_____	(1)
10. Copy the design		_____	(1)

TOTAL SCORE   _____

Level of Consciousness [subjective observation]: Alert   Drowsy   Stupor   Coma

V. DEPRESSION

A. Presentation: apathy, depressed affect, sleep or appetite changes, psychomotor retardation

B. Assessment: The Beck Depression Inventory is a useful tool for assessing depression. Patients with moderate to severe depression always warrant psychiatric referral. All patients should be asked about suicidal/homicidal ideation, intent, and plan and can be referred to a psychiatrist on this basis alone. The risk of suicide in HIV patients, especially those with a previous history of attempted suicide, may be high due to organic changes and depression.

C. A word about suicide: Risk of suicide should be assessed whenever you are working with depressed patients. The most important factors to consider are these:

1. Plan: Is it detailed, lethal, and available?
2. Mental state: Is the patient hopeless? Conversely, does the patient have a new, unexplained peace with no change in circumstance?
3. Precipitating crisis: Has the patient recently experienced a significant loss?

VI. BECK DEPRESSION INVENTORY (BDI)

The BDI is a useful measure of symptoms of depression as specifically indicated by alteration in mood, negative self-concept, regressive and self-punishing wishes, changes in activity level, and movement toward passivity. The inventory contains 21 multiple-choice items, answered in terms of self-evaluated severity. The range of possible scores is 0 to 63 based on a simple sum of values (0 to 3) from each item. A cutoff score of 16 may indicate an individual at risk for having a depressive disorder. The complete kit of the BDI, including the manual and 25 record forms, is $46.00 and is available from The Psychological Corporation, Order Service Center, P.O. Box 839954, San Antonio, TX 78283-3954 (phone: 1-800-228-0751).

VII. GUIDELINES FOR TREATMENT OF NEUROPSYCHOLOGICAL SYMPTOMS

A. Anxiety symptoms: In the absence of cognitive difficulties, judicious use of benzodiazepines is most useful.
B. Depression: With either functional depression (defined as major depression in the *Diagnostic and Statistical Manual of Mental Disorders*—4th edition [*DSM-IV*]) or organic mood disorder (i.e., depression secondary to neurological changes), antidepressants are indicated. Generally speaking, the tricyclics with the least side effects of anticholinergic activity, orthostatic changes, and sedation are indicated. These include desipramine (Norpramin) and nortriptyline (Pamelor) in doses of 50 to 125 mg, by mouth (po), every day (qd). Amitryptyline (Elavil) is particularly troublesome. Fluoxetine (10-20 mg po qd) can also be used.
C. Cortical dementia: If aggression, agitation, hostility, or paranoia is part of the symptom complex, neuroleptics are the drug of choice. Haldol Halperidol (Haldol) in doses of 2 to 30 mg po qd, and Trilafon perphenazine (Trilafon) in doses of 6 to 48 mg po qd, can be very helpful. Patients with HIV disease are highly susceptible to dystonias and extrapyramidal symptoms and may need anticholinergics such as trihexyphenidyl HCL (Cogentin; 0.5-2 mg po qd) or benzotropine mesylate (Artane; 2-5 mg po qd). These drugs may not control aggression or agitation, and other measures may be needed. Generally, a psychiatric consultation is necessary to determine if augmentation would help. Benzodiazepines,

BUSPAR (a 5-HT1A blocker), anticonvulsants, and antidepressants may at times be very useful.

D. Subcortical dementia: Methylphenidate (Ritalin) in doses of 5 to 40 mg, po, qd, is clearly the drug of choice for patients with subcortical dementia.

VIII. TIPS FOR MANAGING ADC

The capacity to remember general concepts and specific details greatly enhances patients' abilities to organize their lives. The ability to remember events through the passage of time allows individuals to feel that they can assert a level of personal control over their quality of life and experience of living. The ADC continuum includes a progressive loss of these capabilities.

When the patient experiences these losses, feelings of frustration and stress can quickly enhance deficits and act to decrease even further the individual's daily ability to use functions that allow him or her to engage in a participatory lifestyle.

The use of memory cues and organizational aides may assist individuals to compensate for these deficits and help to preserve their freedom. Competencies should be supported to the fullest extent possible.

Suggestions for the Patient

Use a calendar.

Post notes as reminders (turn off the stove, lock the door).

Use an automated pillbox.

Keep an appointment book.

Maintain consistency in room setup.

Develop daily routines.

Carry a notepad.

Do one task at a time.

Stay mentally active in nonstressful ways.

Stay well rested.

Schedule appointments in the early part of the day.

Practice stress reduction techniques.

Involve friends and/or family to help remember appointments.

Suggestions for Caregivers

Give simple instructions for task completion.

Break tasks into their component parts.

Ask yes or no questions rather than open questions.

Minimize unnecessary choices; give positive direction.

Speak simply.

Give the patient ample time to respond.

Arrange for a life-call button if necessary.

11

Housing and Home Care

The housing and supportive home care component of these guidelines outlines a continuum of responsible housing options for people with HIV disease. Everyone should have access to safe, affordable, and permanent housing that enhances one's quality of life.

Evaluating patients' housing in relationship to their physical health and level of functioning is an important but often overlooked task. Individuals living in unstable or inappropriate housing relative to their ability to care for themselves are likely to deteriorate physically. This may be due to an inability to meet needs for nutrition, hygiene, safety, treatments, and rest. In addition, living in an inappropriate environment can diminish a patient's hope, sense of self-worth, and will to follow through on treatment recommendations. You, as the provider, can play an important role in assessing the appropriateness of a patient's environment and assisting the patient to access housing, home-based support, or residential care more appropriate to his or her needs.

Most patients prefer to live in an environment where their independence is maximized. Referral to appropriate visiting nurse, hospice care, or AIDS service organizations often allows patients to avoid institutionalization. Patients who are homeless and ill often need medical documentation from you to be able to access housing programs. Shelters are inappropriate environments for patients who are ill because they do not offer the support needed.

Housing Guidelines

IMPORTANCE OF EVALUATING PATIENT HOUSING STATUS

- The optimal housing environment for maximizing a patient's physical and mental health is one that is stable, within the patient's financial means, and provides the most autonomy a patient can physically, mentally, and behaviorally negotiate.
- Determine whether or not the patient's present housing situation is appropriate for his or her current medical condition and whether or not the patient will be able to remain in the current housing environment. Because finding appropriate alternative housing may be practically and emotionally difficult and time-consuming, it is best to raise the issue and monitor the setting before it becomes a problem.
- The questions in Table 11.1 will help you evaluate patient safety and risk of becoming homeless. If you determine that a patient's environment is unsafe, referral to a case manager, social worker, or continuing care nurse is indicated. In some situations, patients can be maintained at home by bringing in home care services such as visiting nurses and home health aides. At other times alternative housing options must be pursued.

If answers to the questions in Table 11.1 indicate that the patient is in need of supports to remain in the home, consider referral to a local home health agency. If the answers indicate that the patient is in inadequate housing or in danger of losing housing, consider referral to the hospital social services department or to a local AIDS service organization for case management or housing advocacy.

NOTE: For a more complete picture of a patient's living situation, it is helpful to speak with family members, friends, and others involved in the patient's care.

Housing Options

NOTE: Exploring patient desires about supported living arrangements prior to serious illness provides you with a basis for assisting patients with making difficult choices later.

TABLE 11.1 Evaluating Present Housing Situation

Safety Issues

Is the patient living on the street?

Is the patient actively using drugs? Are others in the patient's environment actively using drugs?

What is the patient's physical ability to negotiate his or her environment? (e.g., steps or stairways)

What is the patient's mental status? Can he or she remember to eat, lock the door, turn off the stove, and so on? Is there someone else available to provide supervision if necessary?

Is anyone in the patient's environment physically abusive?

Ability to Care for Self in Present Environment

Does the patient's level of pulmonary and ambulatory functioning permit the patient to function adequately within his or her environment?

What level are the patient's activities of daily living (ADLs, e.g., cooking, dressing, bathing, etc.)?

Does the patient have the energy levels to manage these activities? Is there anyone in the patient's environment who can assist with these tasks if needed?

Does the patient have any children that he or she is caring for? Does the patient have the physical and mental ability to care for them adequately? Is additional support needed?

Is the patient actively using substances? How is this affecting the patient's ability to care for himself or herself?

Would a referral to a case manager, social worker, or continuing care provider be helpful?

Financial Issues

Does the patient have the financial ability to remain in his or her present housing? Is the patient paying more than 50% of his or her income for rent or a mortgage?

Has the patient's economic situation recently changed due to illness-related loss of employment? Is it likely to in the near future?

Is the patient in imminent danger of eviction?

Has the patient applied for all financial benefits that he or she is entitled to?

Would a referral to a case manager, social worker, or continuing care provider be helpful?

Socioeconomic Issues

Does the patient live with others or alone? What relationship does the patient have to others in the household? Are household members available to provide emotional or practical support?

Are other members of the household aware of the patient's diagnosis? Is the patient welcome to remain?

Does the patient have privacy? How disruptive to the household will it be to bring in services such as home care?

Where does the patient live in relation to family members and friends? How isolated is the patient? Does the patient wish to relocate to be closer to family?

Is anyone in the home physically or mentally abusive? Is anyone in the household actively using drugs?

Would a referral to a case manager, social worker, or continuing care provider be helpful?

INDEPENDENT HOUSING

If a patient has the ability to care for himself or herself or has the support to be maintained in an independent environment, this option may be appropriate. Factors that impinge on the feasibility of this arrangement include changes in financial, mental, and physical status. Awareness of these changes allows you to make referrals before the situation becomes a crisis.

HOUSING SUBSIDIES

Federally funded rental assistance programs, such as Section 8, can be applied for through local housing authorities. There is often a waiting list, so patients in need of financial assistance should be encouraged to apply as early as possible. Some AIDS service organizations also have programs to help meet housing costs or have information about accessing other housing programs available in your area.

LOW-INCOME HOUSING

Low-income patients can contact local housing authorities for information about available low-income housing units and for applications. Local AIDS service organizations may be able to assist with this process.

SCATTERED-SITE INDEPENDENT APARTMENTS

Some AIDS organizations run scattered-site apartment programs for people with HIV. These apartments are subsidized and often have support staff available. Criteria for acceptance into these programs vary. In most instances, applicants will not be accepted if they are actively using illicit drugs.

SUPPORTIVE AIDS RESIDENCES

Residential programs offering different levels of support and supervision are available. Usually, these programs are congregate settings with shared kitchen, bathroom, and common areas. Bedrooms are either single or shared. Services that may be available include 24-hour supervision, on-site support groups, recreational activities, volunteer support, and so on. Programs offering 24-hour supervision may be ideal for patients who do not need a medical setting but who are unsafe in an independent setting.

STEP DOWN HOUSING

Step down housing offers support to addicts with HIV who are working on maintaining their recovery. This consists of independent, subsidized units staffed by drug treatment counselors.

CHRONIC CARE FACILITIES

For patients who need 24-hour care but do not meet the criteria for a skilled nursing facility, referral to a chronic care facility may be indicated. This can be considered when adequate support to maintain the patient at home is not available. Some chronic care hospitals may have specialized AIDS units.

NURSING HOMES

Patients who need extensive nursing care and cannot be maintained at home may require placement in a skilled nursing or intermediate care facility. Institutions vary in their ability to meet the complex needs of AIDS patients, such as the provision of intravenous therapies, methadone, rehabilitation, or other services.

RESIDENTIAL HOSPICES

Patients with late-stage HIV disease who are ready for palliative care rather than more aggressive forms of management could benefit from hospice placement. Making this decision is a difficult process that requires the patient to come to terms with death.

> *NOTE:* Shelters are generally not an acceptable option for patients who are ill. Most shelters require residents to be outside all day long and wait in lines for daily readmission; they do not offer an environment in which patients are able to care for themselves adequately or receive services. Every effort should be made to find an alternative.

Home Care Options

PERSONAL SUPPORT NETWORK

You can play a facilitative role in structuring the involvement of a patient's friends and family members as part of a care team. Offering education to caregivers can alleviate their anxieties and enhance their comfort level in caring for the patient. Bringing caregivers together to develop a care plan and a specific schedule can be key to keeping a patient at home.

VOLUNTEER SUPPORT

AIDS service organizations, church groups, and other community groups offer volunteer services. These include individuals who offer emotional support, companionship, and assistance with chores, such as housecleaning, shopping, cooking, transportation, baby-sitting, respite care, and other activities. Volunteers can be integral members of a care team.

PERSONAL CARE ATTENDANT

In some states, reimbursement is available for patients to hire someone, including a friend or family member, to assist with nonmedical care. The home care section of the state health department can guide you in accessing this resource. A physician order is necessary.

HOMEMAKER

Home health agencies, such as visiting nurse associations, provide homemaking services, including cooking, cleaning, and shopping for patients too ill to carry out these activities. A physician order is necessary.

HOME HEALTH AIDE

Nonnursing hands-on care is available through home health agencies. Extended hours of coverage may be possible, depending on insurer approval and staff availability. A physician order is necessary.

VISITING NURSE

If a patient's stability is in question or if specific treatments are required, a visiting nurse referral is appropriate. The nurse can administer medications, assess a patient's condition, evaluate needs, educate members of the care team, and coordinate care with other disciplines. A physician order is necessary.

HOME INFUSION

Patients in need of infusion therapies can receive them at home through private home infusion companies or their local home health agencies. Nurses administer treatments, monitor patients, or teach patients and care team members to administer the medications themselves. A physician order is necessary.

IN-HOME HOSPICE

In-home hospice uses an interdisciplinary approach to address physical, psychosocial, and spiritual needs of the patient, family, and significant others. Patients who qualify for hospice can receive specialized services and additional hours of care. A physician order is necessary.

> *NOTE:* Exploring patient wishes regarding long-term and immediate preferences for care will make difficult decisions easier later, especially if a patient becomes incapable of communicating his or her desires. Bring in resources such as a visiting nurse and hospice services as early as possible. You will need to check with insurers, Medicaid, or the agencies themselves to determine patient eligibility for services.

12

Financial Assistance

Many people with AIDS find themselves suddenly unable to manage financially due to loss of income, insurance, and other job benefits. The individual's ability to access quality health care, maintain housing, and have an active social life may all be abruptly threatened. This threat compounds the stress of already having to manage the many physical problems associated with HIV disease. Others who have been able to maintain only a marginal existence may suddenly find their illness prevents them from surviving in their usual ways on the street or in shelters, relying on friends or family members, or living from hand to mouth in other ways. In either circumstance, financial problems can significantly contribute directly or indirectly to a patient's physical health.

Local, state, and federal programs provide numerous forms of financial assistance. *Patients should apply for all programs for which they may be eligible. Many of these programs will require you to extensively document your patients' disability for them to qualify.*

The importance of helping patients achieve financial stability in the face of an unpredictable, life-threatening illness cannot be stressed enough. *Your patients will be relying on you to respond promptly and in depth to all requests for disability verification from agencies providing financial assistance.*

The following section provides information useful to you in helping your patients get the benefits to which they are entitled.

Public Financial Assistance Programs Available to People With HIV

I. GENERAL ASSISTANCE (CITY/TOWN WELFARE)

NOTE: Many states do not have general assistance programs. Regulations regarding general assistance programs vary widely from state to state. The following is a general guide to the application process.

A. Eligibility

1. Means test: A person must be without sufficient money to meet basic living expenses.

2. Residency: Generally, persons must reside within the town where they apply for benefits. Usually, homeless people can apply within the town in which they were living at the time they became homeless or within the town in which they reside that has a shelter.

B. Benefits

1. Most localities will provide several days of emergency food and shelter while a general assistance application is pending.

2. Needs covered by general assistance usually include rent or shelter and food. A subsidy to meet daily living expenses may be provided.

3. General assistance recipients in some localities are eligible for medical benefits.

C. Application Process

1. Generally, applicants are expected to apply in person at the welfare office in their town. If a client is too disabled to apply in person he or she may be able to arrange for a social worker to come to his or her home or make arrangements for a telephone interview.

2. Time frames for response to applications and for appeals are determined by geographic region.

3. Applicants must bring identification and proof of address to their first visit. They will usually need to provide additional financial documentation on subsequent visits.

4. Employable applicants in some states need to participate in workfare. If your patient is too disabled to work, he or she may need to bring medical documentation to attest to this.

5. If an applicant is denied benefits, he or she is entitled to apply for a hearing. Time limits for this vary by locality. Before being terminated from general assistance, a person must be given written notice.

6. Additional information on benefits and rules governing general assistance should be available from your state, regional, or local general assistance office.

D. Application Assistance: AIDS service organizations, legal aid offices, and community action programs may be able to assist patients with the application or appeals process.

Social Security Disability Insurance (SSDI) and Supplemental Security Income (SSI)

I. PROGRAM DEFINITION

A. SSDI is a federal benefits program administered through the Social Security Administration (SSA) that pays income on the basis of how much money a person has paid into the system throughout his or her work history. Eligibility is based solely on disability. SSDI recipients are eligible for Medicare after 2 years of receiving benefits.

B. SSI is a federal benefits program administered through the SSA and has no work history requirement. Eligibility is based on a means test in conjunction with disability. Most SSI recipients are eligible for Medicaid (state medical benefits). However, they must apply separately for this.

II. DEFINITION OF DISABILITY

A. For the purposes of the SSA, a person is considered disabled if he or she has a severe physical or mental impairment or combination of impairments that prevents him or her from working for a year or more or that is expected to result in death. This applies to the person's ability to maintain any gainful employment, not just employment in his or her field.

B. In some instances, a person may be eligible for benefits on the basis of the disability of another family member, such as a minor child or recently deceased spouse.

III. DOCUMENTING DISABILITY

A. *Your patient's ability to receive benefits directly hinges on your comprehensive and detailed evaluation of his or her disability. If benefits are denied due to incomplete medical information, the patient must wait at least 6 months before being reevaluated for benefits.*

B. Applicants for both SSDI and SSI are required to provide extensive documentation of the severity of their disability. Documentation of disability *must* be supplied by a physician. To expedite your patient's application, provide as much detailed information as you can. HIV status or an AIDS diagnosis, in and of itself, is not sufficient. Completion of the presumptive disability form, available from the SSA, will *greatly* expedite this process.

C. The SSA requires documentation of CD4 cell counts, complete physical exam findings, opportunistic infections, additional signs and symptoms, weight loss in relation to percentage of baseline weight, and lab data. Common manifestations of HIV considered when evaluating claims include the following:

1. Symptoms of HIV infection

   a) Low energy, fatigue, generalized weakness

   b) Fever, night sweats

   c) Dyspnea on exertion

   d) Weight loss

   e) Persistent cough

   f) Persistent diarrhea

   g) Depression, anxiety

   h) Forgetfulness, loss of concentration, slowness of thought

   i) Other symptoms, such as headache, anorexia, nausea, vomiting, or symptoms that may be side effects from prescribed medications

2. Signs of HIV/AIDS infection

   a) Documented weight loss

   b) Documented fevers

   c) Lymphadenopathy

   d) Oral thrush/hairy leukoplakia

   e) Abnormal skin conditions

   f) Asthenia

   g) Depression/mental changes

   h) Central or peripheral neurological deficit

3. Laboratory abnormalities

   a) Leukopenia, lymphopenia, anemia, thrombocytopenia

   b) Elevated erythrocyte sedimentation rate

   c) Elevated serum globulin

   d) Depressed helper CD4 cell count

   e) Inverted helper/suppressor ratio

   f) Positive HIV antibody test (including confirmatory test)

   g) X-ray or imaging changes

   h) Microbiology and pathology reports

   i) Other indicators of immune status, such as elevated β2-microglobulins, detectable p24 antigen, and so on

4. Description of functional limitations

    a) Limitation in ability to bathe, dress, or take public transportation independently

    b) Limitation in ability to perform specific activities, such as carrying a 10-pound bag of groceries up a flight of stairs

    c) Limitation in ability to stand and/or walk for 6 to 8 hours per day or sit for 6 to 8 hours per day

    d) Limitation in ability in any other areas that might affect the claimant's potential for work-related activities

Be sure also to include information on other conditions the patient may have that are not related to HIV, such as lupus, diabetes, and scoliosis. The disability determination is based on cumulative physical and mental conditions.

D. SSDI and SSI recipients periodically need to recertify their eligibility for continuing benefits. During a recertification process, you will be asked to provide recent documentation of continued disability.

E. If a patient's condition improves and he or she wishes to return to work, provisions exist under which he or she may continue to receive at least partial benefits while working. More information on this is available from the SSA.

IV. APPLYING FOR DISABILITY

A. The formula for figuring out which of these two benefit programs your patients are eligible for is cumbersome and detailed. Encourage patients to apply for both. The SSA will determine which program's eligibility criteria are met by each patient. In some instances, patients will be eligible to receive benefits under both programs.

B. Typically, applications take up to 3 months to process. Also, there is a 6-month waiting period from the date of disability until the start-up of SSDI benefits. Encourage your patients to begin the application process immediately so they do not lose out on any money to which they are entitled.

C. Applicants must bring an extensive amount of information with them to begin their claims process. They should call ahead to find out everything they will need. Be sure they have your correct name, phone number, and address to bring with them when they apply.

D. Attached is a tips sheet you can photocopy and give to your patients to assist them in applying for Social Security benefits. To find out the phone number and location of your local Social Security office call 1-800-772-1213.

Tip Sheet for Persons Applying
for Social Security Benefits

You may be eligible for both Social Security Disability (SSDI), which is based on your work history, and Supplemental Security Income (SSI), which is based on how much money and property you own. Apply for both programs.

It usually takes 2 to 3 months for a final decision after you hand in your application. Even if it takes a few months to begin receiving benefits, if you are eligible, the government owes you money from the date you apply, *so apply for benefits as soon as you can.*

If you do not feel well enough to go to the Social Security office, you can call and ask them to take your application by telephone.

The application process can be confusing. Call local AIDS organizations for help.

When you apply for benefits, you will be asked for the following information:

- Social security number
- Work history, including dates
- Earnings information from this year and last year. (It is helpful to have a pay stub, W-2 form, or an income tax return.)
- Medical condition, with *details* of your physical/emotional/mental condition. Write a list of everything that has been bothering you in the past several months, including when each problem started. They do *not* have to be related to HIV.
- Names, addresses, and phone numbers of doctors, hospitals, clinics, and so on
- Hospitalization dates; other information about your medical history
- Family responsibilities and dependents, including social security numbers and ages of any children you have
- Education background/special training you have/special skills

About 2 or 3 months after you apply, you will receive either a letter telling you how much money you are getting or a letter telling you why you will not be getting any money. If you do not get a letter from Social Security after 3 months, call and ask about the status of your case.

If you disagree with Social Security's decision, you have a right to appeal (ask them to change their decision). Your local Legal Aid Society or AIDS service organization may be able to help you appeal. You have 60 days to file an appeal after receiving notice about your claim.

Other Financial Assistance Programs

MEDICAID

Medicaid is a federal medical assistance program administered in partnership with state governments. States are required by federal law to cover some services, such as hospitalizations and physician care, for those who are eligible. States have flexibility in determining other services that they will cover. Some states will pick up payments for an individual's insurance premium under the Consolidated Omnibus Budget Reconciliation Act (COBRA) rather than reimburse for services directly. States are also allowed to place limits on required services.

Medicaid pays claims for medically necessary services for eligible individuals. Payment is usually made directly to the providers. Providers must be Medicaid certified to receive payment.

Many Medicaid beneficiaries qualify automatically as a result of their eligibility for cash assistance through programs such as SSI and Aid to Families With Dependent Children (AFDC). However, states have a great deal of latitude in determining who is eligible for Medicaid, and some states have set Medicaid income eligibility levels below those for SSI. Patients on Medicaid must be reviewed periodically to redetermine their eligibility for this program.

Persons with HIV disease qualify for Medicaid in two basic ways:

- They become disabled (see previous disability definition) as a result of their illness and deplete their resources, thus qualifying as medically needy. In many states, qualifying for SSI is sufficient to make a patient eligible for Medicaid.
- They may fall into a group that automatically qualifies for Medicaid, such as a group receiving AFDC or low-income pregnant women.

Medicaid is administered by each state through a single state agency, usually the department responsible for welfare and social service programs or the health department. This department can be contacted for more information.

MEDICARE

Individuals who receive SSDI automatically receive Medicare after 2 years. Medicare covers costs associated with hospitalization. Patients will also receive information from Medicare on how to apply for Part B coverage at this time. This covers physician and outpatient costs. A premium for this care will be deducted from the patient's Social Security check.

CONSOLIDATED OMNIBUS BUDGET RECONCILIATION ACT (COBRA)

Anyone working for an employer with 20 or more employees who leaves his or her job has the right to continue in his or her employer's group health plan for a period of at least 18 months. Premiums may not rise more than 2% above the normal rate for a healthy employee. The employee can pay the former employer monthly and must be offered the same coverage provided active employees.

AID TO FAMILIES WITH DEPENDENT CHILDREN (AFDC)

This is a means-tested federal financial assistance program for families with minor children. Eligibility for this program is based solely on financial need. Families receiving AFDC are automatically qualified to receive Medicaid benefits. It is not necessary to be disabled. Application is made through local welfare offices.

FOOD STAMPS

Many people receiving benefits such as general assistance, AFDC, or SSI are also eligible for food stamps. Food stamps are coupons that are redeemable at supermarkets and other stores for food and household goods. Separate application at the local welfare office is necessary.

AIDS DRUG ASSISTANCE PROGRAM

Subsidies are available under a federal program to help pay for drugs related to AIDS treatment. This program is administered at the state level. Each state determines income eligibility requirements and what treatments are covered. In many instances, patients who work will still be able to meet the income requirements. Most states cover antiviral drugs such as zidovudine (ZDV), didanosine, and zalcitabine. Many states cover medications commonly used for prophylaxis, such as rifabutin and Bactrim. Some states also cover nutritional supplements and vitamins. Contact your state health department or local AIDS service organization to find out how to apply for this program.

PRIVATE INSURANCE

If a patient has private insurance, the insurance company must treat HIV infection as any other illness or disability and provide what the contract mandates. If the patient did not have health insurance before testing HIV positive, it is very difficult to get coverage because most insurance companies screen applicants for HIV. In the event that the patient cannot receive insurance coverage, he or she may contact state and local agencies that provide medical and financial assistance or the state insurance commission.

LIFE INSURANCE BUYOUTS

There are now a proliferation of companies who will buy a patient's life insurance policy if it has a cash value. This allows patients to benefit from their life insurance policies before they die. This can be an excellent source of income for people with HIV, but they should be careful in assessing the terms of the buyout.

13

Legal Issues

HIV and the Law

Although people with HIV are primarily concerned with obtaining appropriate medical care, they must contend with many nontreatment issues to sustain a decent quality of life. They may experience discrimination in housing or the workplace, breaches of the confidentiality of their HIV status, and concern about whether their wishes regarding medical treatment and property disposition will be followed.

A person living with HIV or AIDS can ensure himself or herself a better quality of life by taking some steps to prevent legal problems from occurring. People often feel better when they take control of their lives. Learning one's legal rights (see Appendix 13–A) and planning for disability can help create that important sense of control.

Some of the situations confronting persons with HIV have legal remedies, and there are attorneys throughout the country who are willing and able to represent people with HIV (see Appendix 13–B).

These are examples of situations in which your patient could benefit from having an attorney:

- Your patient's HIV status has been disclosed without the patient's permission to the patient's employer or landlord.
- Your patient is fired by his or her employer after submitting insurance claims for HIV treatments.
- Your patient wants a friend or same-sex partner to make medical decisions for him or her if he or she becomes unable to make or communicate such decisions. The patient is concerned that his or her family will make the decisions instead of the friend or the partner.
- Your patient cannot be discharged from the hospital because no nursing home will accept the patient or because no home health care agency will provide services for the patient.
- Your patient is a single parent with end-stage AIDS who has not arranged for the guardianship of her or his minor children.
- The Social Security Administration has denied your patient's application for disability benefits, and his or her precarious financial position is undermining his or her health.

HIV Testing and Confidentiality

Many states have laws requiring that a person give his or her informed consent to the administration of a HIV test before the test is administered. There are usually some limited emergency exceptions to that strict rule.

Many states also prohibit the disclosure of confidential HIV-related information, except in very limited circumstances, without the permission of the person who was tested for HIV or who has HIV. Some states may impose on medical professionals a duty to warn third parties of likely danger. No involuntary disclosure about a patient's HIV status should be made without first seeking ethical and legal opinions.

Legal Protection Against
HIV-Related Discrimination

People with HIV and those whom others perceive to be at risk for contracting HIV often encounter discrimination in areas such as housing, employment, and insurance. HIV and AIDS are considered disabilities under various federal and state laws that prohibit discrimination against people who have disabilities. These antidiscrimination laws offer varying degrees of protection from the prejudiced attitudes and unsupported fears of others, which often result in HIV-related discrimination.

What follows is a brief description of some of the legal protections available to people who are subjected to HIV-related discrimination. This is not an exhaustive list of the legal options that may be available in a particular case. If the patient has experienced HIV-related discrimination, he or she should obtain professional legal assistance. Keep in mind that each antidiscrimination law has a deadline by which a person must initiate legal action. Contacting a private attorney or legal assistance organization as soon as possible after a discriminatory experience is recommended.

- The Americans With Disabilities Act of 1990 (ADA) is a federal law that forbids discrimination against persons with disabilities in employment, public accommodations, public services, and other aspects of American life. The law requires the reasonable accommodation of an otherwise qualified person with a disability.
- The Vocational Rehabilitation Act of 1973 prohibits discrimination against people with HIV, or those perceived to be at risk of having HIV, by federal agencies and federal contractors. Section 504 of the act also prohibits discrimination by any program or activity that receives federal funds, such as schools that receive educational grants or hospitals and nursing homes that accept Medicaid and Medicare. The act requires the agency, contractor, program, or activity to make reasonable accommodations to the handicaps of otherwise qualified persons, such as employees, patients, and students, who would otherwise not be able to benefit from or participate in the program or activity.
- The Employee Retirement Income Security Act (ERISA) of 1974 prohibits the discharge of, or discrimination against, an employee if the purpose of the discrimination is to deprive the employee of health or pension benefits.
- The Fair Housing Amendments Act of 1988 prohibits discrimination on the basis of handicap in the purchase of housing or in the rental of housing in a building with more than four units.
- Employees working under a collective bargaining agreement may have an additional source of protection. Almost all union contracts place limits on the arbitrary dismissal of an employee and authorize arbitration of disputes over employee discipline and discharges.
- Most states have human rights laws that prohibit discrimination against persons with disabilities in employment, housing, public accommodations, and other areas.

Maintaining Health Insurance

Most employers that sponsor group health plans must offer employees and their families health plan coverage beyond the employee's date of employment.

Under the Consolidated Omnibus Budget Reconciliation Act (COBRA), most employers with 20 or more employees must allow employees who leave their jobs to continue their health care coverage for at least 18 months beyond their last day of employment. Coverage can be extended for a total of 29 months if the Social Security Administration decides that the employee was disabled when the employee left work.

Some states mandate programs that supplement COBRA and extend the continuation of coverage rules to small-group health plans. The cost of the continued coverage to the employee is the group rate plus a small administrative fee. States may use Medicaid funds to pay the continuation coverage premiums of people who leave their jobs because of HIV disease.

BENEFITS PROGRAMS

There are numerous programs available to provide benefits to persons with disabilities. If one of your patients is denied benefits, an attorney can represent the patient at hearings or in court.

Life Planning

Life planning involves preparing written instructions concerning medical care and the disposition of property. Life planning enables a person to make sure that wishes are honored even if he or she becomes unable to give direction on desired treatment. It also prevents conflict about who should inherit any possessions after death. These are some of the documents used in life planning (the names and functions of these planning tools may vary from state to state):

- A *living will* is a document in which a patient can tell his or her doctor whether he or she wants to be kept alive by life support systems, such as ventilators and feeding tubes, if the patient becomes gravely ill.
- A patient can appoint a spouse, relative, or friend to be a *substitute medical decision maker*. This person can advise the doctor about the patient's wishes regarding medical treatments when the patient is no longer able to communicate those wishes.
- A patient can give broad responsibility to another person (the attorney-in-fact) to handle financial affairs by giving that person a *power of attorney*.
- A *will* is a document in which instructions are given for the distribution of property after death. If a will is not written, property will be distributed to the

spouse, children, and blood relatives according to a formula contained in state law. A patient can nominate a guardian for minor children in his or her will, but that nomination may not be enforceable.

- A *conservator* is a person who is appointed by the court to handle the personal and/or financial affairs of an adult who is unable to manage his or her affairs or to take care of himself or herself.

Appendix 13–A: State Laws

STATE LAWS CONCERNING REPORTING OF NAMES OF PERSONS TESTING POSITIVE
FOR HIV ANTIBODIES; INFORMED-CONSENT REQUIREMENTS FOR HIV ANTIBODY
TESTING; CONFIDENTIALITY OF INFORMATION CONCERNING HIV STATUS; ANONY-
MOUS TESTING; QUARANTINE; MANDATORY TESTING OF PRISONERS AND PERSONS
CHARGED WITH OR CONVICTED OF CRIMES; CRIMINAL LAWS CONCERNING TRANS-
MISSION OF HIV AND DEFENDANTS WITH HIV; AND RELATED STATUTES*

Key to Using the State-By-State Information

This appendix is divided as follows.

Reporting. All states require reporting of AIDS cases as defined by the
Centers for Disease Control. This section lists only laws and regulations relating
to the requirements for reporting of HIV-positive people to a state agency.

Informed Consent. This section lists statutory supplements to common-
law-informed consent requirements, specific exceptions under which informed
consent for HIV testing is not necessary, and penalties for violations of the
statutory informed-consent requirements. Statutes cited in the categories concerning informed consent refer specifically to HIV unless otherwise noted.

Confidentiality. This section lists state laws concerning confidentiality of
HIV test results, statutes authorizing anonymous testing, exceptions to nondisclosure provisions, and penalties for violations of the confidentiality provisions. Most states allow sharing of a patient's HIV status between health care
workers when necessary for the care and treatment of the patient. These
statutes are not listed under "Exceptions to Nondisclosure," although they may
be subject to abuse.

Affirmative Duty to Disclose. This section lists statutes creating an affirmative duty to disclose HIV infection.

---

*This statutory compilation was prepared by Sharon L. Irving while working as a legal
intern with the National Lawyers Guild AIDS Network under grants from the Berkeley
Law Foundation, the Ken Bryan Fund, and the Steven Richter Fellowship Fund/NEFIR
and is based on the work of Thomas W. Tierney. We gratefully acknowledge the
assistance of the Intergovernmental Health Policy Project, Gerald Roemer, and Rachel
A. Mariner.

Quarantine. This section lists public health laws relating to quarantine that either are or may be applicable to people with HIV.

Mandatory Test. This section lists laws regarding nonconsensual testing in the criminal context.

Transmission Crime. This section lists statutes concerning the criminal consequences of HIV transmission.

If no entry is noted for a category, the state does not have a statute under the heading.

Many statutes listed in this appendix do not refer to HIV directly but instead mention sexually transmitted diseases (STDs) or communicable diseases (CDs). These references are noted parenthetically, along with relevant state laws and regulations concerning the classification of HIV infection as an STD or as a CD.

Further information about state regulations and laws can be obtained from the state organizations listed in Appendix 13–B. Most of these offices are very helpful, and practitioners are urged to contact them concerning recent changes in state regulations.

Alabama

Reporting: Ala. Code § 22-11A-14 (Supp. 1989) (STDs*) (names)

Confidentiality: Ala. Code § 22-11A-22 (Supp. 1989) (STDs*)

    Exceptions to nondisclosure: Ala. Code § 22-11A-38 (Supp. 1989) (STDs*) (health care/emergency workers; funeral directors, school superintendents; anyone for whom there is a "foreseeable, real, or probable risk of transmission")

    Penalties for wrongful disclosure: Ala. Code § 22-11A-22 (Supp. 1989) (STDs*) (misdemeanor)

Quarantine: Ala. Code § § 22-11A-18, -23 to -32 (Supp. 1989) (STDs*) ("to protect public health")

Mandatory testing: Ala. Code § 22-11A-17 (Supp. 1989) (STDs*) (all convicted prisoners upon entering and upon release from jail or prison); *id.* § 22-11A-37 (STDs*) (when there is reasonable cause to believe an inmate [pre- or postconviction] is infected with an STD)

Transmission crimes: Ala. Code § 22-11A-21(c) (Supp. 1989) (STDs*) (misdemeanor)

---

*Alabama classifies HIV infection as a sexually transmitted disease. Rules of State Board of Health, Division of Disease Control, § 420-4-1-.03 (1987).

Alaska

Reporting: No HIV reporting.
Confidentiality: Alaska Stat. § 09.25.120 (1989) (generally)

Arizona

Reporting: Ariz. Admin. Dig. R9-6-604, -701 (1990) (names)
Statutory informed-consent requirement: Ariz. Rev. Stat. Ann. § 36-663(A) (Supp. 1990)

Exceptions to informed consent: Ariz. Rev. Stat. Ann. § 36-663(B) (Supp. 1990) (body parts for medical research; medical research when test subject cannot be identified; autopsies for public health purposes; emergency situations; persons without capacity to consent when test deemed medically necessary)

Penalties for violations of informed consent: Ariz. Rev. Stat. Ann. § § 36-666, -677 (Supp. 1990) (misdemeanor and civil penalties)

Confidentiality: Ariz. Rev. Stat. Ann. § 36-664(A) (Supp. 1990) (CDs and HIV)

Anonymous testing statute: Ariz. Rev. Stat. Ann. § 36-136(H)(15) (Supp. 1990)

Exceptions to nondisclosure: Ariz. Rev. Stat. Ann. § 13-1415 (Supp. 1990) (victims of sexual offense); id. § 32-1457 (health care or emergency workers); id. § 32-1860 (sexual or needle-sharing partners); id. § 36-664

Penalties for wrongful disclosure: Ariz. Rev. Stat. Ann. § § 36-666, -667 (Supp. 1990) (misdemeanor and civil penalties)

Quarantine: Ariz. Rev. Stat. Ann. § 36-136(H)(1) (Supp. 1990) (CDs)

Mandatory testing: Ariz. Rev. Stat. Ann. § 36-669 (Supp. 1990) (prisoners if there is "reasonable belief that the person is infected with HIV and is a health threat to others"); id. § 13-1415 (persons convicted of sexual offense involving "significant exposure" of bodily fluids and after request by victim)

Arkansas

Reporting: Ark. Stat. Ann. § 20-15-904(b) (Supp. 1989) (names, unless tested anonymously)

Statutory informed-consent requirement: Ark. Act No. 289 (1991) *to be codified* as Ark. Stat. Ann. § 20-15-905

    Exceptions to informed consent: Ark. Act No. 289 (1991) § § 2, 3 *to be codified* as Ark. Stat. Ann. § 20-15-905(b), (c) (exposure of health care worker, medical judgment of physician)

Confidentiality: Ark. Stat. Ann. § 20-15-904(c) (Supp. 1989)

    Exceptions to nondisclosure: Ark. Stat. Ann. § 16-82-101(c) (Supp. 1989). (Where a defendant in criminal prosecution is subject to mandatory testing, a potentially exposed person may request to be informed of test results.)

Affirmative duty to disclose: Ark. Stat. Ann. § 20-15-903 (Supp. 1989). ("Any person who is found to have HIV infection shall, prior to receiving any health care services of a physician or dentist, advise such physician or dentist that the person has HIV infection"; violation is a misdemeanor.)

Mandatory testing: Ark. Stat. Ann. § 16-82-101(b)(1) (Supp. 1989) (persons charged with sexual assaults or with prostitution, after finding of "reasonable cause")

Transmission crimes: Ark. Stat. Ann. § 5-14-123(b) (Supp. 1989) (felony)

California

Reporting: No HIV reporting.

Statutory informed-consent requirement: Cal. Health & Safety Code § 199.22 (West Supp. 1990)

Confidentiality: Cal. Health & Safety Code § § 199.20, .21 (West Supp. 1990)

    Exceptions to nondisclosure: Cal. Health & Safety Code § § 199.24, .25, .27, .97 (West Supp. 1990) (health care workers, sexual or needle-sharing partners, guardian, conservator authorization for testing for reasons of incompetency or for persons under 12 years of age, assault accusers, assaulted peace officers)

    Penalties for wrongful disclosure: Cal. Health & Safety Code § 199.22 (West Supp. 1990) (civil remedy plus misdemeanor)

Mandatory testing: Cal. Health & Safety Code § § 199.96, .97 (West Supp. 1990) (persons charged with sexual assaults on peace officer, after finding of "probable cause" that transfer of bodily fluids took place); Cal. Welf. & Inst. Code § 1768.9 (West Supp. 1990) (juveniles under control of Youth Authority); Cal. Penal Code § 1524.1 (West Supp. 1992) (on request of any crime victim, felony or misdemeanor); *id.* § § 7511-7512.5 (prisoners, either after exposure of other inmates or law enforcement employees to bodily fluids or after manifestations of symptoms of AIDS or ARC); *id.* § 1202.1 (persons convicted of sexual assault victims notified); *id.* § 1202.6 (persons convicted of prostitution of second time); Cal. Code Regs. tit. 22, div. 2, ch. 8 (1991) (general provisions concerning testing of inmates in correctional facilities)

Transmission crimes: Cal. Penal Code § 647f (West Supp. 1990) (felony to continue working as prostitute after knowledge of HIV infection); Cal. Penal Code § 12022.85 (West Supp. 1990) (3-year enhancement of sentence for each conviction of rape, statutory rape, sodomy, or oral copulation after knowledge of HIV infection)

Colorado

Reporting: Colo. Rev. Stat. § § 25-4-1402(1),(2); 25-4-1405(7)(b)(I) (Supp. 1991) (names, unless tested as part of research experiment)

Statutory informed-consent requirement: Colo. Rev. Stat. § 25-4-1405(8) (a) (1989)

    Exceptions to informed consent: Colo. Rev. Stat. § 25-4-1405(8)(a) (1989 and Supp. 1991) (after exposure of health care worker or employee of department of corrections; prisoners; patients without capacity to consent; seroprevalence surveys when test subjects cannot be identified; patients in custody of Department of Corrections)

Confidentiality: Colo. Rev. Stat. § § 25-4-1404 (1989 and Supp. 1991) (Public Health Reports)

    Exceptions to nondisclosure: Colo. Rev. Stat. § 25-4-1404(1)(c) (Supp. 1991) (health care workers); *id.* § 18-3-415 (accusers of sexual penetration; exception not applicable to public health reports)

    Penalties for wrongful disclosure: Colo. Rev. Stat. § 25-4-1409 (Supp. 1991) (misdemeanor)

Quarantine: Colo. Rev. Stat. § § 25-4-1406, -1407 (1989 and Supp. 1991) ("as a last resort"; "least restrictive measures")

Mandatory testing: Colo. Rev. Stat. § 18-3-415 (Supp. 1991) (defendants bound over for trial after preliminary hearing for sexual offense involving sexual penetration; results may be revealed to accuser)

Transmission crimes: Colo. Rev. Stat. § 18-7-201.7 (Supp. 1991) (felony to commit act of prostitution with knowledge of infection); *id.* § 18-7-205.7 (felony to patronize a prostitute with knowledge of infection)

Connecticut

Reporting: No HIV reporting

Statutory informed-consent requirement: Conn. Gen. Stat. § 19a-582 (1991)

 Exceptions to informed consent: Conn. Gen. Stat. § 19a-582 (1991) (when subject unable to consent and test deemed medically necessary; medical research; after "significant" occupational exposure; autopsies; in correctional facilities when medically necessary; in correctional facilities where inmate's behavior poses risks to others; court order; insurance purposes)

 Penalties for violations of informed consent: Conn. Gen. Stat. § 19a-590 (1991) (civil remedies)

Confidentiality: Conn. Gen. Stat. § 19a-583 (1991)

 Exceptions to nondisclosure: Conn. Gen. Stat. § 19a-583(a) (1991) (health care or emergency workers; prison employees); *id.* § 19a-584 (sexual or needle-sharing partners)

 Penalties for wrongful disclosure: Conn. Gen. Stat. § 19a-590 (1991) (civil remedies)

Mandatory testing: Conn. Gen. Stat. § 19a-582 (1991) (prisoners for treatment purposes or if behavior of inmate poses significant risk of transmission to another inmate or has resulted in significant exposure of another inmate and no reasonable alternative exists)

Delaware

Reporting: Del. State Board of Health, Regulations for the Control of Communicable and Other Disease Conditions § 7.412 (1990) (no names except from Blood Bank of Delaware)

Statutory informed-consent requirement: Del. Code Ann. tit. 16, § 1202(a) (Supp. 1990)

Exceptions to informed consent: Del. Code Ann. tit. 16, § 1202(c) (Supp. 1990) (after exposure of health care workers); *id.* § 703 (STDs*) (on order of director of division of public health "when necessary to protect the public health"); *id.* § 708 (STDs*) prenatal testing of pregnant women)

Penalties for violations of informed consent: Del. Code Ann. tit. 16, § 1204 (Supp. 1990) (civil remedies)

Confidentiality: Del. Code Ann. tit. 16, § 711, § 1203 (Supp. 1990)

Exceptions to nondisclosure: Del. Code Ann. tit. 16, § 1203(a)(3) (Supp. 1990) (health care workers)

Penalties for wrongful disclosure: Del. Code Ann. tit. 16, § 1204 (Supp. 1990) (civil remedies)

Quarantine: Del. Code Ann. tit. 16, § § 703 to 705 (Supp. 1990) (STDs*) (as last resort)

---

*Del. Code Ann. tit. 16, § § 1202(c)(5), 1203(a)(9) (Supp. 1990); authorize exceptions to informed consent and nondisclosure pursuant to the chapter on sexually transmitted diseases.

District of Columbia

Reporting: No HIV reporting

Confidentiality: D. C. Code Ann. § § 6-2805, 6-117 (1989) (HIV and CDs*)

Exceptions to nondisclosure: D. C. Code Ann. § 6-117(b)(1)(B) (1989) (CDs*) (when court determines that disclosure is "essential to safeguard the physical health of others" or would afford evidence probative of guilt or innocence in criminal prosecution)

Quarantine: D. C. Code Ann. § § 6-119 to -123 (1989) (CDs*)

---

*The District of Columbia classifies HIV infection as a communicable disease (telephone conversation between Thomas Tierney and Jean Tapscott of the AIDS Program of the District of Columbia Commission on Public Health, July 1990).

Florida

Reporting: Fla. Stat. Ann. § 384.25(3) (West Supp. 1991) (no names)

Statutory informed-consent requirement: Fla. Stat. Ann. § 381.609(3)(a) (West Supp. 1991)

Exceptions to informed consent: Fla. Stat. Ann. § 381.609 (West Supp. 1991) testing of deceased by medical examiner; bonafide medical emergency; medical judgment of physician; "significant" exposure of medical personnel; hospitalized infant where medically indicated); *id.* § 381.6105 (blood products or human tissue received from out-of-state health care facility; blood products or human tissue received from health care provider for reference testing or processing and results reported back to same provider; unrevoked anatomical gift by deceased or incompetent donor); *id.* § 384.31 (prenatal testing of pregnant women for STDs*)

Confidentiality: Fla. Stat. Ann. § § 381.609(3)(f), 384.29 (West Supp. 1991) (HIV and STDs*)

Anonymous testing statute: Fla. Stat. Ann. § 381.609(4)(c) (West Supp. 1991)

Exceptions to nondisclosure: Fla. Stat. Ann. § 381.609 (West Supp. 1991) (health care workers; foster or adoptive parents; sexual assault accusers); *id.* § 455.2416 (sexual or needle-sharing partners); *id.* § 960.003 (sexual assault accusers)

Penalties for wrongful disclosure: Fla. Stat. Ann. § 381.609(6)(b) (West Supp. 1991) (misdemeanor)

Contact tracing: Fla. Stat. Ann. § 384.26 (West Supp. 1991)

Quarantine: Fla. Stat. Ann. § § 384.27-.288 (West Supp. 1991) (STDs*) (as last resort)

Mandatory testing: Fla. Stat. Ann. § 796.08(3) (West Supp. 1991) (prostitutes and persons "injuring" peace officer where nature of injury is such as to result in transmission); *id.* § 960.003 (persons charged with any sexual offense involving transmission of bodily fluids and on accuser's request); *id.* § 381.609 (persons convicted of prostitution or charged with sexual battery where a "blood sample is taken from the defendant voluntarily or pursuant to court order for any purpose"); *id.* § 384.32 (STDs*) (prisoners)

Transmission crimes: Fla. Stat. Ann. § 384.24 (West Supp. 1991) (STDs*) (misdemeanor); *id.* § 796.08(5) (separate misdemeanor penalties for prostitution after knowledge of positive test result)

---

*Florida classifies HIV infection as a sexually transmitted disease. See Fla. Stat. Ann. § 384.23 (West Supp. 1991).

Georgia

Reporting: Ga. Code Ann. § 31-22-9.2(b) (Harrison 1990) (no names)

Statutory informed-consent requirement: Ga. Code Ann. § 31-22-9.2(c)
(Harrison 1990)

> Exceptions to informed consent: Ga. Code Ann. § 31-17A-2 (Harrison
> Supp. 1990). (When necessary to protect public health, public health
> authorities may petition court for order to test person suspected of
> HIV infection if person refuses to be tested.) Ga. Code Ann. §
> 31-22-9.2(c) (Harrison Supp. 1988) (minor or incompetent with
> consent of parent or guardian; health care emergency; medical
> judgment of physician)

Confidentiality: Ga. Code Ann. § 24-9-40.1 (Harrison 1990) (generally); Ga.
Code Ann. § 24-9-47(b) (Harrison Supp. 1990)

> Exceptions to nondisclosure: Ga. Code Ann. § 24-9-47(g), (h), (i)
> (Harrison 1990) (sexual or needle-sharing partner or child, disclosure
> by Department of Human Resources to persons reasonably believed
> to be at risk of infection from disclosed patient, health care workers);
> id. § 17-10-15(e)(1) (victims of "AIDS transmitting crime"); Ga. Code
> Ann. § 24-9-47 (Michie 1991) (proceedings regarding person alleged
> to be mentally ill, mentally retarded, alcoholic, drug dependent
> pursuant to Title 29); id. § 42-1-7 (prisoners)

> Penalties for wrongful disclosure: Ga. Code Ann. § 24-9-47(o), (u)
> (Harrison 1990) (misdemeanor for intentional or knowing disclosure
> of confidential information; no penalty for unintentional violation if
> precautions taken to avoid risks of disclosure unless due to gross
> negligence or wanton and willful misconduct)

Quarantine: Ga. Code Ann. § 88-1204 (1986 and Supp. 1988)

Mandatory testing: Ga. Code Ann. § 17-10-15 (Harrison 1990) (after guilty
verdict or plea, or plea of nolo contendere to charge of "AIDS transmitting
crime"); id. § 15-11-35.1 (juveniles convicted of "AIDS transmitting crime")
id. § 42-5-52.1 (inmates in state prison system)

Transmission crimes: Ga. Code Ann. § 16-5-60 (Harrison 1990). (Donation
of blood, blood products, other bodily fluids or parts; prostitution; needle
sharing; oral or anal sex after knowledge of HIV infection and without disclosure of HIV infection to partner are felonies.)

Hawaii

Reporting: Haw. Rev. Stat. § § 325-2, -104 (Supp. 1989) (no names)

Statutory informed-consent requirement: Haw. Rev. Stat. § 325-16 (Supp. 1989)

>   **Exceptions to informed consent:** Haw. Rev. Stat. § 325-16(b) (Supp. 1989) (anatomical gifts; research in which test subject cannot be identified; Department of Health anonymous testing; testing ordered by a third party where written consent obtained for release of results to that third party; medical judgment of physician; exposure of health care workers)

>   **Penalties for violations of informed consent:** Haw. Rev. Stat. § 325-16(d) (Supp. 1989) (civil penalty of at least $1,000)

Confidentiality: Haw. Rev. Stat. § § 325-101 (Supp. 1989)

>   **Exceptions to nondisclosure:** Haw. Rev. Stat. § 325-101 (Supp. 1990), *amended by* S.B. 140, 16th Leg., Reg. Sess. (1991) (medical emergency; to or by Department of Health when no person can be identified and disclosure necessary to protect public health and well-being; by Department of Health to medical personnel, organ banks, courts, etc., by confidential communication to enforce existing law; child's records of Department of Human Services and child protective services team consultants; by Department of Health to natural parents, guardian ad litem of child, court, adoptive parents, foster parents, or medical personnel responsible for care or treatment of child; to health care insurer in order to obtain reimbursement, provided that patient offered opportunity to make reimbursement directly; by patient's health care provider to another provider for purpose of continued treatment; pursuant to a court order after showing of good cause after judge reviews records in camera)

>   **Penalties for wrongful disclosure:** Haw. Rev. Stat. § 325-102 (Supp. 1989) (civil penalty of at least $1,000 plus costs)

Idaho

Reporting: Idaho Code § 39-606 (Supp. 1990) (classified diseases*) (names)

Statutory informed-consent requirement: Idaho Code § 39-4303A (1985) (generally)

Exceptions to informed consent: Idaho Code § 39-4303A (Supp. 1990) (after "significant" exposure of health care or emergency workers and patient incapable of giving consent)

Confidentiality: Idaho Code § 39-610 (Supp. 1990)

Exceptions to nondisclosure: Idaho Code § 39-604 (Supp. 1990) (sexual assault accusers); *id.* § 39-4303A (health care or emergency workers)

Penalties for wrongful disclosure: Idaho Code § 39-606 (Supp. 1990) (misdemeanor)

Contact tracing: Idaho Code § 39-610 (Supp. 1990) (of those "who, in the judgment of health authorities, have been exposed to HIV")

Mandatory testing: Idaho Code § 39-604(1) (Supp. 1990) (all prisoners upon admission and upon release)

Transmission crimes: Idaho Code § 39-608 (Supp. 1990). (Sharing needles or engaging in sexual activity after knowledge of HIV infection and without full disclosure to partner is a felony.)

---

*Idaho includes HIV infection as a classified disease for reporting purposes (telephone conversation between Thomas Tierney and Fritz Dixon of the Idaho Department of Health and Welfare AIDS Program, July 1990).

Illinois

Reporting: Ill. Admin. Code tit. 77, § 693.30 (1990) (no names); Ill. Ann. Stat. ch. 111½, para. 7351 (AIDS registry)

Statutory informed-consent requirement: Ill. Ann. Stat. ch. 111½, para. 7304 (Smith-Hurd Supp. 1991)

Exceptions to informed consent: Ill. Ann. Stat. ch. 111½, paras. 7307(a) to (c), 7308 (Smith-Hurd Supp. 1991) (after exposure of health care or emergency workers; anonymous research; medical judgment of physician)

Penalties for violations of informed consent: Ill. Ann. Stat. ch. 111½, para. 7312 (Smith-Hurd Supp. 1988) (misdemeanor)

Confidentiality: Ill. Ann. Stat. ch. 111½, paras. 7309, 7408 (Smith-Hurd Supp. 1991) (HIV and STDs*)

Anonymous testing statute: Ill. Ann. Stat. ch. 111½, paras. 7306, 7408 (Smith-Hurd Supp. 1991) (HIV and STDs*)

Exceptions to nondisclosure: Ill. Ann. Stat. ch. 111½, para. 7309 (Smith-Hurd Supp. 1991) (spouses; health care or emergency workers; foster parents); *id.* para. 22.12a (schools); *id.* para. 7408(a)-(c) (appropriate state agencies; subpoena; warrant for isolation/quarantine)

Penalties for wrongful disclosure: Ill. Ann. Stat. ch. 111½, paras. 7312, 7408 (Smith-Hurd Supp. 1988) (HIV and STDs*) (misdemeanor)

Contact tracing: Ill. Ann. Stat. ch. 111½, para. 7405 (Smith-Hurd 1988) (STDs*)

Quarantine: Ill. Ann. Stat. ch. 111½, paras. 7406-7407 (Smith-Hurd 1988) (STDs*) (mandatory counseling, isolation)

Mandatory testing: Ill. Ann. Stat. ch. 38, para. 1005-5-3(g), (h) (Smith-Hurd Supp. 1991) (persons convicted of sexual assault, prostitution, or hypodermic syringe offense)

Transmission crimes: Ill. Ann. Stat. ch. 38, para. 12-16.2 (Smith-Hurd Supp. 1991) (felony)

---

*Illinois classifies HIV infection as a sexually transmitted disease. See Ill. Ann. Stat. ch. 111, para. 7403 (Smith-Hurd Supp. 1988), Ill. Admin. Code tit. 77, § 693.20(a).

Indiana

Reporting: Ind. Code Ann. § 16-1-9.5-2(b), (c)(2) (West Supp. 1991) (names, unless tested anonymously)

Statutory informed-consent requirement: Ind. Code Ann. § 16-1-9.5-2(a) (West Supp. 1991)

Confidentiality: Ind. Code Ann. § 16-1-9.5-7 (West Supp. 1991) (CDs*)

Exceptions to nondisclosure: Ind. Code Ann. § 16-1-10.5-11.5 (West Supp. 1991) (CDs*) (sexual or needle-sharing partners); *id.* § 16-1-45-7 (CDs*) (emergency workers); *id.* § 35-38-1-10.6 (sexual assault victims and prostitution "victims"); *id.* § 16-1-9.5-9 (funeral directors)

Penalties for wrongful disclosure: Ind. Code Ann. § 16-1-9.5-7(b) (West Supp. 1991) (CDs*) (misdemeanor)

Quarantine: Ind. Code Ann. §§ 16-1-9.5-4, 16-1-10.5-15 to -20 (West Supp. 1991) (HIV and CDs*)

Mandatory testing: Ind. Code Ann. § 35-38-1-10.5(a) (West Supp. 1991) (persons convicted of sexual assault, prostitution, or hypodermic syringe offense; *id.* § 35-38-2-2 (for same persons as condition of parole)

Transmission crimes: Ind. Code Ann. § 35-38-1-7 (West Supp. 1991). (Knowledge of HIV-positive status is an aggravating factor in determining sentence for sexual assault and prostitution offenses.)

---

*Indiana classifies HIV infection as a communicable disease (telephone conversation between Thomas Tierney and Jerry Burkman of the Indiana State Board of Health AIDS Program, July 1990).

Iowa

Reporting: Iowa Code Ann. § 141.8 (West 1989) (no names)

Statutory informed-consent requirement: Iowa Code Ann. § 141.22 (West 1989 and Supp. 1991)

> Penalties for violations of informed consent: Iowa Code Ann. § 141.24 (West Supp. 1991) (civil remedies)

Confidentiality: Iowa Code Ann. § 141.10, .23 (West 1989 and Supp. 1991)

> Anonymous testing statute: Iowa Code Ann. § 141.4 (West 1991)

> Exceptions to nondisclosure: Iowa Code Ann. § 141.6(3)(b) (West Supp. 1991) (sexual or needle-sharing partners); *id.* § 141.23(c) (West 1989) (health care workers); *id.* § 141.25 (funeral directors)

> Penalties for wrongful disclosure: Iowa Code Ann. § 141.24 (West Supp. 1991) (civil remedies)

Mandatory testing: Iowa Code Ann. § 246.514 (West Supp. 1991) (persons committed to correctional institutions who engage in high-risk behavior)

Kansas

Reporting: Kan. Stat. Ann. § 65-6002 (1990) (demographic data, no names)

Confidentiality: Kan. Stat. Ann. § 65-6002(c), -6003(b) (1990)

> Anonymous testing statute: Kan. Stat. Ann. § 65-6007 (1990)

> Exceptions to nondisclosure: Kan. Stat. Ann. § 65-6004(a), (b) (1990) (health care workers, emergency personnel, law enforcement officers, spouses or partners); *id.* § 22-2913(d) (victims of crimes involving transmission of bodily fluids); *id.* § 65-2438 (funeral directors)

> Penalties for wrongful disclosure: Kan. Stat. Ann. § 65-6005 (1990) (misdemeanor)

Mandatory testing: Kan. Stat. Ann. § 22-2913(c) (1990) (upon conviction of crime that "involved or may have involved the transmission of bodily fluids")

Kentucky

Reporting: Ky. Rev. Stat. Ann. § 211.180(1)(b) (Michie/Bobbs-Merrill Supp. 1991) (no names)

Statutory informed-consent requirement: Ky. Rev. Stat. Ann. § 214.625(2), (5) (Michie/Bobbs-Merrill 1991); *id.* § 311.291

> Exceptions to informed consent: Ky. Rev. Stat. Ann. § 214.625(2), (3) (Michie/Bobbs-Merrill 1991) (under general consent; emergency situations)

Confidentiality: Ky. Rev. Stat. Ann. § § 214.420, .625(5)(c) (Michie/Bobbs-Merrill 1991)

> Anonymous testing statute: Ky. Rev. Stat. Ann. § 214.625(6)(c) (Michie/ Bobbs-Merrill 1991)

> Exceptions to nondisclosure: Ky. Rev. Stat. Ann. § 214.625(5)(c) (Michie/Bobbs-Merrill 1991) (health care workers; pursuant to court order); *id.* § 331.282 (spouses; sexual partners with whom patient has cohabited for more than 1 year)

> Penalties for wrongful disclosure: Ky. Rev. Stat. Ann. § 214.990(6) (Michie/Bobbs-Merrill 1991) (STDs*) (fine of between $50 and $100)

Mandatory testing: Ky. Rev. Stat. Ann. § 197.055 (Baldwin 1991) (prisoners, if prisoner either engaged in high-risk behavior or was involved in a situation with prison employee that could result in transmission); *id.* § 529.090 (Baldwin Supp. 1991) (persons convicted of prostitution)

Transmission crimes: Ky. Rev. Stat. Ann. § 311.990(25) (Michie/Bobbs-Merrill 1990) (felony to donate organs, skin, or other tissue after knowledge of HIV infection); *id.* § 529.090 (Baldwin Supp. 1991) (felony to commit prostitution by engaging in sexual activities likely to transmit HIV after knowledge of HIV infection and knowing that transmission through sexual activity is likely)

---

*Kentucky classifies HIV infection as a sexually transmitted disease. See Ky. Rev. Stat. Ann. § 214.410 (Baldwin Supp. 1991).

Louisiana

Reporting: No HIV reporting

Statutory informed-consent requirement: La. Rev. Stat. Ann. § 40:1299.40
(West Supp. 1990) (generally)

> Exceptions to informed consent: La. Rev. Stat. Ann. § 40:1299.40 (West
> Supp. 1990). (After exposure of health care workers, tests may be
> conducted on blood previously drawn without consent, but consent
> is still needed to draw new blood for testing.)

Confidentiality: La. Rev. Stat. Ann. § 40:1299.142(B) (West Supp. 1990)
(donors at blood banks)

> Exceptions to nondisclosure: La. Rev. Stat. Ann. § 40:1099(A)(1) (West
> Supp. 1990) (emergency workers); *id.* § 40:1099.1 (corpses); *id.* §
> 40:1299.142(B)(4) (funeral directors; by blood banks to physician)

> Penalties for wrongful disclosure: La. Rev. Stat. Ann. § 40:1299.145
> (West Supp. 1990) (fine up to $2,000)

Transmission crimes: La. Rev. Stat. Ann. § 40:43.5 (West Supp. 1990)
(felony to expose another to HIV through sexual contact)

Maine

Reporting: Me. Rev. Stat. Ann. tit. 22, § 1011(3) (Supp. 1989) (no names)

Statutory informed-consent requirement: Me. Rev. Stat. Ann. tit. 5, §
19203-A (1989)

> Exceptions to informed consent: Me. Rev. Stat. Ann. tit. 5, § § 19203-A
> (4), 19203-C (1989 and Supp. 1990) (after "significant" exposure of
> health care/emergency workers and court review)

> Penalties for violations of informed consent: Me. Rev. Stat. Ann. tit. 5,
> § 19206 (1989). (civil remedies plus penalties up to $5,000)

Confidentiality: Me. Rev. Stat. Ann. tit. 5, § § 19203 (1989 and Supp. 1990)

Anonymous testing statute: Me. Rev. Stat. Ann. tit. 5, § 19203-B (1989)

> Exceptions to nondisclosure: Me. Rev. Stat. Ann. tit. 5, § 19203-A(4),
> 19203-C (1989) (health care or emergency workers)

> Penalties for wrongful disclosure: Me. Rev. Stat. Ann. tit. 5, § 19206
> (1989) (civil remedies plus penalties up to $5,000)

Maryland

Reporting: Md. Health-Gen. Code Ann. § 18-207 (1990) (no names)
Statutory informed-consent requirement: Md. Health-Gen. Code Ann. §
18-336(b) (1990), *amended by* Md. H.B. 194, 1991 Md. ALS 535
 Confidentiality: Md. Health-Gen. Code Ann. § § 18-207, -213 (1990),
amended by Md. H.B. 194, 1991 Md. ALS 535
    Exceptions to nondisclosure: Md. Health-Gen. Code Ann. § 18-213
    (1990) (health care workers or emergency workers; law enforcement
    officers) *id.* § 18-337(b) (sexual or needle-sharing partners)
    Penalties for wrongful disclosure: Md. H.B. 194, 1991 Md. ALS 535 (civil
    cause of action in some circumstances)
Mandatory testing: Md. Health-Gen. Code Ann. § 18-338 (1990) (inmates
after exposure of correctional facilities employee)
Transmission crimes: Md. Health-Gen. Code Ann. § 18-601.1 (1990)
(felony)

Massachusetts

Reporting: No HIV reporting
Statutory informed-consent requirement: Mass. Ann. Laws ch. 111, § 70F
(Law. Co-op. Supp. 1991)
    Penalties for violations of informed consent: Mass. Ann. Laws ch. 111,
    § 70F (Law. Co-op. Supp. 1989) (civil penalties)
Confidentiality: Mass. Ann. Laws ch. 111, § 70F (Law. Co-op. Supp. 1989)
    Exceptions to nondisclosure: Mass. Ann. Laws ch. 111, § 111C (Law.
    Co-op. Supp. 1989) (emergency workers)

Michigan

Reporting: Mich. Comp. Laws Ann. § 333.5114 (West Supp. 1990) (names)
Statutory informed-consent requirement: Mich. Comp. Laws Ann. §
333.5133(2) (West Supp. 1991)
    Exceptions to informed consent: Mich. Comp. Laws Ann. § 333.5123
    (West Supp. 1991) (prenatal testing of pregnant women but only if

woman consents); *id.* § 333.5133(12), (13) (after exposure of health care worker if patient is informed about possibility of such test upon admission to health care facility; patient unable to consent)

Confidentiality: Mich. Comp. Laws Ann. § 333.5131(1) (West Supp. 1991)

Anonymous testing statute: Mich. Comp. Laws Ann. § 333.5133(9) (West Supp. 1991)

Exceptions to nondisclosure: Mich. Comp. Laws Ann. § 333.5131 (West Supp. 1991) (health care workers; sexual or needle-sharing partners; school district employees; foster care agencies); *id.* § 333.20191 (emergency workers); *id.* § 333.2843b (funeral directors)

Penalties for wrongful disclosure: Mich. Comp. Laws Ann. § 333.5131 (8) (West Supp. 1991) (misdemeanor)

Contact tracing: Mich. Comp. Laws Ann. § 333.5114a (West Supp. 1991)

Quarantine: Mich. Comp. Laws Ann. § § 333.5203-.5209 (West Supp. 1991) ("serious communicable diseases or infections")

Mandatory testing: Mich. Comp. Laws Ann. § 333.5129 (West Supp. 1991) (persons convicted of prostitution, criminal sexual conduct, or intravenous use of controlled substances; victims notified if they choose); *id.* § 791.267(2) (all other prisoners tested upon arrival at reception center)

Transmission crimes: Mich. Comp. Laws Ann. § 333.5210 (West Supp. 1991). ("Sexual penetration" after knowledge of seropositivity and without informing partner is a felony.)

Minnesota

Reporting: Minn. R. 4605.7040 (1987) (names)

Statutory informed-consent requirement: Minn. Stat. Ann. § 144.765 (West Supp. 1991*)

Confidentiality: Minn. Stat. Ann. § 144.768 (West Supp. 1991*); *id.* § 13.38 (West 1989) (generally)

Exceptions to nondisclosure: Minn. Stat. Ann. 144.762, .767 (West Supp. 1990*) (emergency workers)

Penalties for wrongful disclosure: Minn. Stat. Ann. § 144.769 (West Supp. 1990*) (misdemeanor); *id.* § § 13.08, .09 (West 1988 and Supp. 1990)

Contact tracing: Minn. Stat. Ann. § 144.4172(4) (West 1989)
Quarantine: Minn. Stat. Ann. § § 144.4173-.4186 (West 1989)

*By their terms, these informed consent and confidentiality statutes are limited to testing after "significant exposure" of emergency workers.

Mississippi

Reporting: Miss. State Dept. of Health, Reportable Diseases 1990-1991 (name and address of person with HIV infection must be reported within 48 hours)
> Exceptions to informed consent: Miss. Code Ann. § 41-41-16 (Supp. 1991) (medical judgment of hospital or physician)

Confidentiality: Miss. Code Ann. § 41-23-30 (Supp. 1991) (STDs*)
> Exceptions to nondisclosure: Miss. Code Ann. § 41-23-1(5) (Supp. 1991) (health care workers); *id.* § 41-23-41 (emergency workers); *id.* § 41-39-13 (funeral directors); Miss. H.B. 592, Reg. Sess., 1991 Miss. Laws 425 (victims of sex offenses)

Quarantine: Miss. Code Ann. § 41-23-27, -29 (Supp. 1991) (STDs*) (any person suspected of being infected shall be examined)
Mandatory testing: Miss. H.B. 592, Reg. Sess., 1991 Miss. Laws 425 (all persons convicted of sex offenses sentenced to state penal institution)

*Mississippi classifies HIV infection as a sexually transmitted disease. See Mississippi State Department of Health 1990 List of Reportable Diseases.

Missouri

Reporting: Mo. Ann. Stat. § 191.653(3) (Vernon Supp. 1990) (names, unless tested anonymously)
Confidentiality: Mo. Ann. Stat. § 191.656(1) (Vernon Supp. 1990)
> Anonymous testing statute: Mo. Ann. Stat. § 191.686 (Vernon Supp. 1990)

> Exceptions to nondisclosure: Mo. Ann. Stat. § 191.656(1)(1)(c), (2)(1) (b), (2)(1)(d), (8)(2)(a), (8)(2)(b) (Vernon Supp. 1990) (adoptive or foster parents; health care workers; sexual partners; emergency workers; funeral directors); *id.* § 191.689 (schools)

Penalties for wrongful disclosure: Mo. Ann. Stat. § 191.656(6) (Vernon Supp. 1990) (civil remedies)

Affirmative duty to disclose: Mo. Ann. Stat. § 191.656(5) (Vernon Supp. 1990) (to any health care professional from whom such person receives services)

Mandatory testing: Mo. Ann. Stat. § 191.659 (Vernon Supp. 1990) (all individuals upon delivery to department of corrections and again before release)

Transmission crimes: Mo. Ann. Stat. § 191.677 (Vernon Supp. 1990). (Creating "grave and unjustifiable risk of infecting another with HIV through sexual or other contact" is a felony.)

Montana

Reporting: Mont. Admin. R. 16.28.204 (1987) (no names)

Statutory informed-consent requirement: Mont. Code Ann. § 50-16-1007 (1991)

> Exceptions to informed consent: Mont. Code Ann. § 50-16-1007(9) (1991) (mental incapacity; medical indications of HIV-related condition; medical judgment of physician; exposure of health care worker)

> Penalties for violations of informed consent: Mont. Code Ann. § 50-16-1007(11) (1991) (misdemeanor)

Confidentiality: Mont. Code Ann. § 50-16-1009 (1991)

> Exceptions to nondisclosure: Mont. Code Ann. § 50-16-529 (1991) (to health care provider, family member, sexual partner when there is "need to know"); id. § 50-16-702 (emergency workers)

> Penalties for wrongful disclosure: Mont. Code Ann. § 50-16-1013 (1991) (civil remedies)

Contact tracing: Mont. Code Ann. § 50-16-1009(3) (1991)

Quarantine: Mont. Code Ann. § 50-18-107 (1991) (for STDs, including AIDS)

Transmission crimes: Mont. Code Ann. § 50-18-112 (1991) (for STDs, including AIDS id. § 50-18-101) (misdemeanor to knowingly expose another to infection)

Nebraska

Reporting: Neb. Rev. Stat. § 71-502.04 (Supp. 1988) (no names)

Statutory informed-consent requirement: Neb. Rev. Stat. § 71-504 (Supp. 1988) (CDs*)

Exceptions to informed consent: Neb. Rev. Stat. § 71-510 (Supp. 1989) (after "significant" exposure of emergency worker)

Penalties for violations of informed consent: Neb. Rev. Stat. § 71-506 (Supp. 1989) (CDs*) (misdemeanor)

Confidentiality: Neb. Rev. Stat. § § 71-503.01, -511 (Supp. 1988 and Supp. 1989) (CDs*)

Exceptions to nondisclosure: Neb. Rev. Stat. § 71-509 (Supp. 1989) (health care or emergency workers)

Penalties for wrongful disclosure: Neb. Rev. Stat. § 71-506 (Supp. 1989) (CDs*) (misdemeanor)

---

*Nebraska classifies HIV infection as a communicable disease (telephone conversation between Thomas Tierney and Virginia Wilkinson of the Nebraska Department of Health AIDS Program, July 1990).

Nevada

Reporting: Nev. Rev. Stat. Ann. § 441A.150 (Michie Supp. 1989) (CDs, including HIV*) (no names)

Confidentiality: Nev. Rev. Stat. Ann. § 441A.220 (Michie Supp. 1989) (CDs*)

Exceptions to nondisclosure: Nev. Rev. Stat. Ann. § 441A.190 (Michie Supp. 1989) (CDs*) (schools); *id.* § 441A.320 (accusers of sexual penetration)

Penalties for wrongful disclosure: Nev. Rev. Stat. Ann. § 441A.430 (Michie Supp. 1989) (CDs*) (misdemeanor)

Quarantine: Nev. Rev. Stat. Ann. § 441A.160, .300 (Michie Supp. 1989)

Mandatory testing: Nev. Rev. Stat. Ann. § 201.356(1) (Michie Supp. 1989) (anyone arrested for prostitution); *id.* § 209.385 (each offender committed to the custody of the department of corrections); *id.* § 441A.320 (upon arrest for a crime involving sexual penetration)

Transmission crimes: Nev. Rev. Stat. Ann. § 201.358 (Michie Supp. 1989) (felony to engage in prostitution after testing positive for HIV); *id.* § 441A.180 (CDs*). (Persons conducting themselves in a manner likely to expose others to disease, after warning from health authority, are guilty of a misdemeanor.)

*Nevada classifies HIV infection as a communicable disease that is sexually transmitted (telephone conversation between Thomas Tierney and Vicki Hamilton of the Nevada State Health Division, Department of Human Resources, July 1990).

New Hampshire

Reporting: N.H. Code Admin. Rules HE-P 300, part HE-P 301 (Rev. Oct. 1, 1990) (no names)

Statutory informed-consent requirement: N.H. Rev. Stat. Ann. § 141-F:5 (1990)

Exceptions to informed consent: N.H. Rev. Stat. Ann. § 141-F:5 (1990) (blood banks; donation of body parts; medical research when test subject cannot be identified; individuals confined to correctional facility or committed to a N.H. hospital; patient incapable of giving consent)

Penalties for violations of informed consent: N.H. Rev. Stat. Ann. § 141-F:11 (1990) (misdemeanor if natural person, felony otherwise)

Confidentiality: N.H. Rev. Stat. Ann. § 141-F:8 (1990)

Exceptions to nondisclosure: N.H. Rev. Stat. Ann. § 141-F:8(IV) (1990) (to health care workers to protect health of patient); *id.* § 141-G:5 ("infectious disease") (emergency workers)

Penalties for wrongful disclosure: N.H. Rev. Stat. Ann. § 141-F:11 (1990) (misdemeanor if natural person, felony otherwise)

Contact tracing: N.H. Rev. Stat. Ann. § 141-F:9 (1990)

Mandatory testing: N.H. Rev. Stat. Ann. § 141-F:5(VI) (Supp. 1990) (persons convicted and confined to correctional facility)

New Jersey

Reporting: N.J. Stat. Ann. § 26:5C-6 (West Supp. 1990) (names, unless tested anonymously)

Confidentiality: N.J. Stat. Ann. § 26:5C-7 (Supp. 1990)
Anonymous testing statute: N.J. Stat. Ann. § 26:5C-6 (West Supp. 1990)
(six sites allowed)
Exceptions to nondisclosure: N.J. Stat. Ann. § 26:5C-8(b)(3) (West
Supp. 1990) (health care workers); *id.* § 26:6-8.2 (funeral directors)
Penalties for wrongful disclosure: N.J. Stat. Ann. § 26:5C-14 (West Supp.
1990) (civil remedies)

New Mexico

Reporting: No HIV reporting
Statutory informed-consent requirement: N.M. Stat. Ann. § 24-2B-2 (Supp.
1990)
Exceptions to informed consent: N.M. Stat. Ann. § 24-2B-5(D) (Supp.
1990) (after exposure of health care workers)
Confidentiality: N.M. Stat. Ann. § 24-2B-6 (Supp. 1990)
Exceptions to nondisclosure: N.M. Stat. Ann. § 24-2B-6(C) (Supp. 1990)
(health care workers)
Quarantine: N.M. Stat. Ann. § 24-1-15 (1986) (for "diseases dangerous to
the public health")

New York

Reporting: No HIV reporting
Statutory informed-consent requirement: N.Y. Pub. Health Law § 2781
(McKinney Supp. 1991)
Exceptions to informed consent: N.Y. Pub. Health Law § 2781
(McKinney Supp. 1991) (when processing human tissue for research
or transplant; research where test subject cannot be identified;
autopsies)
Penalties for violations of informed consent: N.Y. Pub. Health Law §
2783 (McKinney Supp. 1991) (civil penalties plus misdemeanor for
willful violations)
Confidentiality: N.Y. Pub. Health Law § 2782 (McKinney Supp. 1991)

Anonymous testing statute: N.Y. Pub. Health Law § 2781(4) (McKinney Supp. 1991)

Exceptions to nondisclosure: N.Y. Pub. Health Law § 2782(1), (4) (McKinney Supp. 1991) (health care workers; adoptive or foster parents; third party reimbursers; insurers when consent requirements met; employees of division of parole or probation when necessary; medical director of corrections facility when necessary; law guardian representing minor; sexual or needle-sharing partners)

Penalties for wrongful disclosure: N.Y. Pub. Health Law § 2783 (McKinney Supp. 1991) (civil penalties plus misdemeanor for willful violations)

North Carolina

Reporting: N.C. Gen. Stat. § 130A-135 (1990) (names, unless tested anonymously)

Statutory informed-consent requirement: N.C. Gen. Stat. § 130A-148(h) (Supp. 1991)

Exceptions to informed consent: N.C. Gen. Stat. § 130A-148(h) (Supp. 1991) ("when necessary to protect the public health"; minors when parents refuse consent and there is reason to believe that minor is HIV infected or has been sexually abused)

Confidentiality: N.C. Gen. Stat. § 130A-143 (1990)

Exceptions to nondisclosure: N.C. Gen. Stat. § 130A-143, -395 (1990) (health care workers; "when necessary to protect the public health"; funeral directors)

Quarantine: N.C. Gen. Stat. § § 130A-144 to -145 (1990 and Supp. 1991) (CDs)

North Dakota

Reporting: N.D. Cent. Code § 23-07-02.1 (Supp. 1989) (names)

Statutory informed-consent requirement: N.D. Cent. Code § 23-07.5-02 (Supp. 1989)

Exceptions to informed consent: N.D. Cent. Code § 23-07.4-01 (Supp. 1989) (as last resort when person is "danger to public health")

Penalties for violations of informed consent: N.D. Cent. Code § 23-07.05-07 (Supp. 1989) (civil remedies)

Confidentiality: N.D. Cent. Code § 23-07.5-05 (Supp. 1989)

Exceptions to nondisclosure: N.D. Cent. Code § 23-07.5-05(1)(b), (1)(g), (2) (Supp. 1989) (health care workers; embalmers, pursuant to court order)

Penalties for wrongful disclosure: N.D. Cent. Code § 23-07.5-07, -08 (Supp. 1989) (civil remedies, felony)

Quarantine: N.D. Cent. Code § 23-07.4-01 to -02 (Supp. 1989) (as last resort)

Mandatory testing: N.D. Cent. Code § 23-07.5-07 (Supp. 1989) (persons convicted of crime and imprisoned for 15 days or more; persons convicted of designated sexual offenses [sexual assault, rape, "deviate sexual act"] or use of controlled substances, whether imprisoned or not)

Transmission crimes: N.D. Cent. Code § 12.1-20-17 (Supp. 1989) (transfer of bodily fluid after knowledge of HIV seropositivity a felony; affirmative defense if transfer was by sexual activity between consenting adults after full disclosure of the risk of such activity and with the use of an appropriate prophylactic device)

Ohio

Reporting: Ohio Rev. Code Ann. § 3701.24(C) (Anderson Supp. 1990) (names)

Statutory informed-consent requirement: Ohio Rev. Code Ann. § 3701.242 (Anderson Supp. 1990)

Exceptions to informed consent: Ohio Rev. Code Ann. § 3701.242 (Anderson Supp. 1990) (medical emergency; research when tested subject cannot be identified; donated body parts; incarcerated persons on the basis of "good cause"; medical judgment of physician; exposure of health care or emergency worker)

Penalties for violations of informed consent: Ohio Rev. Code Ann. § 3701.244 (Anderson Supp. 1990) (civil remedies)

Confidentiality: Ohio Rev. Code Ann. § 3701.243 (Anderson Supp. 1990)
   Anonymous testing statute: Ohio Rev. Code Ann. § 3701.241(B)(2)
   (Anderson Supp. 1990)

   Exceptions to nondisclosure: Ohio Rev. Code Ann. § 3701.243
   (Anderson Supp. 1990) (sexual partners; health care or emergency
   workers; pursuant to court order); id. § 2907.27(B) (sexual assault
   accusers)

   Penalties for wrongful disclosure: Ohio Rev. Code Ann. § 3701.244
   (Anderson Supp. 1990) (civil remedies)

Mandatory testing: Ohio Rev. Code Ann. § 2907.27(B) (Anderson Supp.
1990) (anyone charged with sexual assault—disclosure to accuser if requested)

Oklahoma

Reporting: Okla. State Board of Health, Regulations for Reporting Cases of
Disease, § § 100 et seq. (names, unless tested anonymously)
   Confidentiality: Okla. Stat. Ann. tit. 63, § 1-502.2 (West Supp. 1991) (CDs*)
   Exceptions to nondisclosure: Okla. Stat. Ann. tit. 63, § 1-502.2(A)(3)
   (West Supp. 1991) (CDs*) (when necessary to protect health and
   well-being of general public); id. § § 1-502.2(A)(4), -502.1(B) (CDs*)
   (health care or emergency workers; funeral directors)

   Penalties for wrongful disclosure: Okla. Stat. Ann. tit. 63, § 1-502.2
   (West Supp. 1991) (CDs*) (misdemeanor plus civil remedies)

Mandatory testing: Okla. Stat. Ann. tit. 63, § 1-524 (West Supp. 1992)
(persons arrested for first or second degree rape, forcible sodomy, intentional
infection, or attempt to intentionally infect with HIV)

Transmission crimes: Okla. Stat. Ann. tit. 21, § 1031(B) (West Supp. 1991)
(felony to engage in prostitution with knowledge of HIV infection); id. § 1192.1
(felony to engage in any activity "with intent to infect or cause to be infected"
another person with HIV)

---

*Oklahoma classifies HIV infection as a communicable disease for the purposes of Okla.
Stat. Ann. tit. 63, § 1-502.2 because HIV infection is "required to be reported pursuant
to" Okla. Stat. Ann. tit. 63, § 1-503.

Oregon

Reporting: Or. Admin. R. 333-18-030(1) (1988) (no names)

Statutory informed-consent requirement: Or. Rev. Stat. § 433.045(1) (Supp. 1990); *id.* § 433.065 (procedures upon exposure of health care worker); Or. Admin. R. § 333-12-265, -266 (1990)

> Exceptions to informed consent: Or. Rev. Stat. § 433.080 (Supp. 1990); Or. Rev. Stat. § 333-12-269 (after "substantial" exposure of health care workers; patients exposed by health care workers)

Confidentiality: Or. Rev. Stat. § 433.045(3) (Supp. 1990); Or. Rev. Stat. § 333-12-270 (1990)

> Exceptions to nondisclosure: Or. Rev. Stat. § 433.075(5) (Supp. 1990) (health care or emergency workers); Or. Rev. Stat. § 333-12-270 (1990) (medical judgment of physician; persons having had a "substantial" exposure whereby identity of HIV-infected individual remains confidential; anatomical gifts)

Mandatory testing: Or. Rev. Stat. § 135.139 (Supp. 1990) (persons convicted of crime where transmission of bodily fluids was likely to have occurred but only if victim requests test and has also submitted to HIV antibody test; victim is then notified of results)

Pennsylvania

Reporting: No HIV reporting

Statutory informed-consent requirement: Pa. Stat. Ann. tit. 35, § 7605 (Purdon Supp. 1991) (generally and as pertains to insurers)

> Exceptions to informed consent: Pa. Stat. Ann. tit. 35, § 7605(g) (Purdon Supp. 1991) (cadaver for use in medical research; medical research when test subject cannot be identified; as needed by insurers who have satisfied consent requirements; medical emergency); *id.* § 7606 ("significant" exposure of health care worker)

Confidentiality: Pa. Stat. Ann. tit. 35, § 7607 (Purdon Supp. 1991)

> Exceptions to nondisclosure: Pa. Stat. Ann. tit. 35, § 7607 (Purdon Supp. 1991) (health care workers; emergency situations; insurer when necessary for reimbursement; funeral directors; agencies responsible for placement and health care of dependent or delinquent youth)

Penalties for wrongful disclosure: Pa. Stat. Ann. tit. 35, § § 7610-11 (Purdon Supp. 1991)

Quarantine: Pa. Stat. Ann. tit. 35, § 521.11 (Purdon 1977) (VDs*)

Mandatory testing: See Pa. Stat. Ann. tit. 35, § 521.8 (Purdon 1977) (VDs*) (any person charged with crime involving lewd conduct or sex offense "may be examined" for VD)

---

*One Pennsylvania trial court has classified AIDS as a venereal disease. See *Commonwealth v. Mason*, 48 Pa. D. & C. 3d 633 (1988).

Rhode Island

Reporting: R.I. Dept. of Health Reg. R23-6-HIV (§ 7) (1989) (no names)

Statutory informed-consent requirement: R.I. Gen. Laws § 23-6-12 (1989)

Exceptions to informed consent: R.I. Gen. Laws § 23-6-14 (Supp. 1990) (postnatal testing of infants; children between the ages of 1 and 13 who appear symptomatic; minors under state care; after "significant" occupational exposure; emergency situations)

Confidentiality: R.I. Gen. Laws § 23-6-17 (1989)

Exceptions to nondisclosure: R.I. Gen. Laws § 23-6-17(b)(iii), (b)(v) (Supp. 1990) (health care workers; persons exposed to bodily fluids of persons "testing positive for AIDS"; persons with whom "AIDS infected" patient is in close and continuous contact if physician perceives danger of transmission and there is reason to believe that infected individual will not inform third party)

Penalties for wrongful disclosure: R.I. Gen. Laws § 23-6-19 (1989) (civil and criminal penalties)

Mandatory testing: R.I. Gen. Laws § 11-34-10 (Supp. 1990) (any person convicted of prostitution); *id.* § 21-28-4.20 (persons convicted of possession of any hypodermic instrument associated with IV drug use); *id.* § 42-56-37 (persons convicted of any crime and committed to adult correctional institution, and again at time of release)

South Carolina

Reporting: S.C. Code Ann. § 44-29-10, -70 (Law Co-op. Supp. 1989) (STDs*) (names); S.C. Reg. 61-21C-F; S.C. Reg. 61-20(1), (6)

Exceptions to informed consent: S.C. Code Ann. § 44-29-230 (Law Co-op. Supp. 1989) (health care workers)

Confidentiality: S.C. Code Ann. § 44-29-135 (Law Co-op. Supp. 1989) (STDs*); S.C. Reg. 61-21G

Exceptions to nondisclosure: S.C. Code Ann. § 44-29-20 (Law Co-op. Supp. 1989) (STDs*) (funeral directors); *id.* § 44-29-135(e) (schools); *id.* § 44-29-136; *id.* § 44-29-146 (physicians and state agencies exempt from liability for disclosure to persons at risk of infection); S.C. Reg. 61-21G, H

Penalties for wrongful disclosure: S.C. Code Ann. § 44-29-140 (Law Co-op. Supp. 1989) (STDs*) (misdemeanor)

Contact tracing/partner notification: S.C. Code Ann. § § 44-29-90, -146 (Law Co-op. Supp. 1990); S.C. Reg. 61-21E, G(1), G(2)(c), G(2)(d), G(5), K(4)(f), K(4)(g), K(4)(h)

Quarantine: S.C. Code Ann. § 44-29-90, -115 (Law Co-op. Supp. 1989) (STDs*); S.C. Reg. 61-21K

Mandatory testing: S.C. Code Ann. § 16-3-740 (Law Co-op. Supp. 1989) (persons convicted of sexual assault in which bodily fluids were exchanged; victims notified); *id.* § 16-15-255 (persons convicted of prostitution or "buggery" in which bodily fluids were exchanged; persons exposed notified); *id.* § 44-29-90 (Law Co-op 1990); *id.* § 44-29-100 (Law Co-op. Supp. 1989) (STDs*); (persons confined or imprisoned may be "examined," isolated)

Transmission crimes: S.C. Code Ann. § 44-29-145 (Law Co-op. Supp. 1990) (felony to knowingly expose another to HIV through exchange of bodily fluids without informing the person of risks)

---

*South Carolina classifies HIV infection as a sexually transmitted disease that is reportable, according to the South Carolina Department of Health's 1990 List of Reportable Diseases.

South Dakota

Reporting: S.D. Codified Laws Ann. § 34-22-12 (1986) (HIV*) (names)

Confidentiality: S.D. Codified Laws Ann. § 34-22-12.1 (Supp. 1991) (CDs*)

Penalties for wrongful disclosure: S.D. Codified Laws Ann. § 34-22-12.2 (Supp. 1991) (CDs*) (misdemeanor)

Quarantine: S.D. Codified Laws Ann. § § 34-22-1 to -4 (1986) (CDs*)

Mandatory testing: S.D. Codified Laws Ann. § 23A-35B-1 (1992). (Upon request of victim of certain violent crimes or law enforcement personnel, the court may order testing of the defendant if there is "probable cause to believe that the defendant committed the offense and that there was an exchange of blood, semen or other body fluid.")

Transmission crimes: S.D. Codified Laws Ann. § § 34-16-1, 2 (1986) (act endangering public health as misdemeanor, release of disease germs as felony); *id.* § 34-22-5 (CDs*) (misdemeanor)

---

*South Dakota classifies HIV infection as a communicable disease. See the South Dakota Department of Health, 1990 List of Notifiable Diseases.

Tennessee

Reporting: Tenn. Dept. of Health, Regulations Governing Communicable Diseases, No. 1200-14-1-.41 (1992). (Names of persons with HIV infection are reportable; anonymous testing abolished.)

Confidentiality: Tenn. Code Ann. § 68-10-113 (Supp. 1990) (STDs*) (applies only to Health Department records)

   Exceptions to nondisclosure: Tenn. Code Ann. § 68-10-113 (Supp. 1990) (STDs*) (pursuant to court order)

   Penalties for wrongful disclosure: Tenn. Code Ann. § 68-10-111 (1987 and Supp. 1990 note) (STDs*) (misdemeanor)

Quarantine: Tenn. Code Ann. § § 68-10-104 to -106, -108 to -110 (1987 and Supp. 1991) (STDs*)

Mandatory testing: Tenn. Code Ann. § 39-13-521 (1991) (convicted individual upon request of victim)

Transmission crimes: Tenn. Code Ann. § § 68-10-107, -111 (1987 and Supp. 1990) (STDs*) (misdemeanor); *id.* § 39-13-516 (1991) (prostitution with knowledge of HIV infection is a felony)

---

*Tennessee classifies HIV infection as a sexually transmitted disease (telephone conversation between Thomas Tierney and Matt Nelson of the Tennessee Department of Health and Environment—Disease Control, July 1990).

Texas

Reporting: Tex. Health & Safety Code Ann. § 81.041(e) (Vernon 1990) (no names)

Statutory informed-consent requirement: Tex. Health & Safety Code Ann. § § 81.102, .105, .106 (Vernon 1992)

> **Exceptions to informed consent:** Tex. Health & Safety Code Ann. § 81.048 (Vernon 1992) (emergency workers); *id.* § 81.107 (health care workers)

> **Penalties for violations of informed consent:** Tex. Health & Safety Code Ann. § 81.102(f) (criminal penalties); *id.* § 81.104 (Vernon 1990) (civil remedies and penalties)

Confidentiality: Tex. Health & Safety Code Ann. § 81.103 (Vernon 1990)

> **Anonymous testing statute:** Tex. Health & Safety Code Ann. § 85.082 (Vernon 1990)

> **Exceptions to nondisclosure:** Tex. Code Crim. Proc. Ann. art. 21.31 (Vernon Supp. 1990) (alleged victims of sexual assault); Tex. Health & Safety Code Ann. § 81.103(b)(8) (1992); *id.* § 81.048 (emergency workers); *id.* § 81.103(b)(5), (b)(7) (health care workers; spouses); Tex. Ed. Code Ann. § 21.933 (teachers)

> **Penalties for wrongful disclosure:** Tex. Health & Safety Code Ann. § 81.103(j) (Vernon Supp. 1990) (criminal penalty); *id.* § 81.104 (civil remedies and penalties)

Contact tracing: Tex. Health & Safety Code Ann. § § 81.048, .051 (Vernon 1990)

Quarantine: Tex. Health & Safety Code Ann. § § 81.083, .151ff (Vernon 1990) (CDs)

Mandatory testing: Tex. Gov't. Code Ann. § 500.054 (Vernon 1990) (Texas Board of Corrections authorized to test inmates); Tex. Code Crim. Proc. Ann. art. 46A.01 (Vernon Supp. 1990) (county may test inmate confined in jail); *id.* art 21.31 (persons indicted for sexual assault; alleged victim notified of results)

Transmission crimes: Tex. Penal Code Ann. § 22.012 (Vernon Supp. 1990) (felony to engage intentionally in conduct reasonably likely to result in transfer of bodily fluids after knowing seropositivity and not informing partner)

Utah

Reporting: Utah Code Ann. § 26-6-3(2) (Supp. 1991) (HIV) (names, unless tested anonymously)
Confidentiality: Utah Code Ann. § § 26-6-20.5, -25a-101 (Supp. 1991)
Anonymous testing statute: Utah Code Ann. § 26-6-3(5) (Supp. 1991)
Exceptions to nondisclosure: Utah Code Ann. § 26-25a-101(2)(b), (2)(h) (Supp. 1991) (peace officers, health care workers)
Penalties for wrongful disclosure: Utah Code Ann. § 26-25a-103 (Supp. 1991) (misdemeanor)
Contact tracing: Utah Code Ann. § 26-6-3(2)(b) (Supp. 1991)
Quarantine: Utah Code Ann. § 26-6-4 (1989) (CDs*)
Mandatory testing: Utah Code Ann. § 64-13-36 (Supp. 1991) ("all state prisoners in July 1989, and upon admission of all who are thereafter committed to the jurisdiction of the department")
Transmission crimes: Utah Code Ann. § 26-6-5 (1989) (CDs) (misdemeanor)

---

*Utah classifies HIV infection as a communicable disease. See Utah Code Ann. § 26-6-3(4) (Supp. 1991).

Vermont

Reporting: No HIV reporting
Statutory informed-consent requirement: Vt. Stat. Ann. tit. 8, § 4724(20)(B) (Supp. 1989) (relating to insurance trade practices only)
Confidentiality: Vt. Stat. Ann. tit. 18, § 1099 (1982) (STDs*)
Exceptions to nondisclosure: Vt. Stat. Ann. tit. 12, § 1705 (Supp. 1989) (by court order)

---

*Vermont classifies HIV infection as a sexually transmitted disease (telephone conversation between Thomas Tierney and Debra Kutzko of the Vermont Department of Health, AIDS Education Program, July 1990).

Virginia

Reporting: Va. Code Ann. § 32.1-36(C) (Supp. 1991) (names)

Statutory informed-consent requirement: Va. Code Ann. § 32.1-37.2 (Supp. 1991)

Exceptions to informed consent: Va. Code Ann. § 32.1-45.1 (Supp. 1991) (after exposure of health care workers)

Penalties for violations of informed consent: Va. Code Ann. § 32.1-27 (Supp. 1991) (generally) (misdemeanor)

Confidentiality: Va. Code Ann. § 32.1-36.1 (Supp. 1991)

Anonymous testing statute: Va. Code Ann. § 32.1-55.1 (Supp. 1991)

Exceptions to nondisclosure: Va. Code Ann. § 32.1-36.1(A)(11) (Supp. 1991) (spouse); *id.* § 32.1-37.1 (funeral directors); *id.* § 32.1-45.1 (health care workers)

Penalties for wrongful disclosure: Va. Code Ann. § 32.1-36.1(B), (C) (Supp. 1991) (civil remedies plus penalty)

Quarantine: Va. Code Ann. § 32.1-43 (Supp. 1991) (generally); *id.* § § 32.1-48.01 to -48.04 (isolation by court order if no other reasonable alternative for reducing risk to public health)

Mandatory testing: Va. Code Ann. § § 32.1-48.01 to -48.04 (Supp. 1991) (by court order for any crime involving sexual assault, all convicted prostitutes)

Washington

Reporting: Wash. Admin. Code § 248-100-076 (1991) (Class IV HIV disease)

Statutory informed-consent requirement: Wash. Rev. Code Ann. § 70.24. 330 (Supp. 1990)

Exceptions to informed consent: Wash. Rev. Code Ann. § 70.24.340 (Supp. 1990) (after "significant" exposure of health care or emergency workers or peace officer); Wash. Admin. Code § 248-100-206(10) (1991)

Penalties for violations of informed consent: Wash. Rev. Code Ann. § 70.24.080 (Supp. 1990) (STDs*) (gross misdemeanor)

Confidentiality: Wash. Rev. Code Ann. § 70.24.105 (Supp. 1990)

Anonymous testing statute: Wash. Rev. Code Ann. § 70.24.105 (Supp. 1991)

Exceptions to nondisclosure: Wash. Rev. Code Ann. § 70.24.105(2)(f), (2)(g), (2)(h), (2)(j) (Supp. 1990) (pursuant to court order; sexual or needle-sharing partners; health care or emergency workers; adoptive or foster parents)

Penalties for wrongful disclosure: Wash. Rev. Code Ann. § 70.24.080 (Supp. 1990) (STDs*) (gross misdemeanor)

Quarantine: Wash. Rev. Code Ann. § § 70.24.022-.034 (Supp. 1990) (STDs*) (as last resort)

Mandatory testing: Wash. Rev. Code Ann. § 70.24.340 (Supp. 1990) (all persons convicted of sexual offense, prostitution, or drug offense associated with hypodermic needles); id. § § 70.24.360-.370 (all jail detainees and prison inmates if their actual or threatened behavior presents "possible risk" to staff)

Transmission crimes: Wash. Rev. Code Ann. § 9A.36.021(d) (Supp. 1991) (assault in the second degree)

---

*Washington classifies HIV infection as a sexually transmitted disease. See Wash. Rev. Code Ann. § 70.24.017 (Supp. 1990).

West Virginia

Reporting: W. Va. Dept. of Health Rule § 64-64-11 (names, unless tested anonymously)

Statutory informed-consent requirement: W. Va. Code § 16-3C-2 (Supp. 1989)

Exceptions to informed consent: W. Va. Code § 16-3C-2(f) (Supp. 1989) (after "possible" exposure of health care or emergency worker or funeral director; persons who "are or may be a danger to the public health" and who are believed by public health officer to be HIV infected)

Penalties for violations of informed consent: W. Va. Code § 16-3C-5 (Supp. 1989) (civil remedies and penalties)

Confidentiality: W. Va. Code § 16-3C-3 (Supp. 1989)

Anonymous testing statute: W. Va. Code § 16-3C-2(c) (Supp. 1989)

Exceptions to nondisclosure: W. Va. Code § 16-3C-3(a)(3), (a)(8), (d) (Supp. 1989) (funeral directors; health care workers; pursuant to court order; sexual or needle-sharing partners while maintaining confidentiality of HIV-infected individuals)

Penalties for wrongful disclosure: W. Va. Code § 16-3C-5 (Supp. 1989) (civil remedies and penalties)

Mandatory testing: W. Va. Code § 16-3C-2(f) (Supp. 1989) (persons convicted of prostitution or sexual abuse/assault)

Wisconsin

Reporting: Wis. Stat. Ann. § 146.025(7)(b) (West 1989 & Supp. 1991) (names, unless tested anonymously)

Statutory informed-consent requirement: Wis. Stat. Ann. § 146.025(2)(a) (West 1989)

Exceptions to informed consent: Wis. Stat. Ann. § 146.025 (West 1989 and Supp. 1991) (organ, sperm, or ova donation; medical research; patient unable to consent; at center for developmentally disabled when medical director determines that patient's conduct poses risks to others; after "significant" exposure of health care worker)

Penalties for violations of informed consent: Wis. Stat. Ann. § 146.025 (8) (West 1989) (civil remedies plus penalties)

Confidentiality: Wis. Stat. Ann. § 146.025(5)(a) (West 1989 and Supp. 1991)

Exceptions to nondisclosure: Wis. Stat. Ann. § 146.025 (West 1989 and Supp. 1991) (health care or emergency workers; funeral directors; sexual or needle-sharing contacts if individual is deceased)

Penalties for wrongful disclosure: Wis. Stat. Ann. § 146.025(9) (West Supp. 1991) (fines to $10,000 and/or imprisonment up to 9 months)

Quarantine: Wis. Stat. Ann. § 143.07 (West 1989) (STDs)

Wyoming

Reporting: Wyo. Stat. § § 35-4-130, -132 (Supp. 1990) (STDs*) (names, unless tested anonymously)

Confidentiality: Wyo. Stat. § 35-4-132(d) (Supp. 1990) (STDs*)

Exceptions to nondisclosure: Wyo. Stat. § § 35-4-132(c), 35-4-133
(Supp. 1990) (STDs*) ("as necessary to protect life and health";
persons who may have had "significant exposure" to STD)

Penalties for wrongful disclosure: Wyo. Stat. § 35-4-130(c) (Supp. 1990)
(STDs*) (misdemeanor)

Quarantine: Wyo. Stat. § 35-4-133 (Supp. 1990) (STDs*) (public health
officer may isolate person "reasonably suspected" of infection with sexually
transmitted disease, provide for examination, and compel treatment)

Mandatory testing: Wyo. Stat. § 35-4-134 (Supp. 1990) (STDs*) (any individual confined or imprisoned "shall be examined" for STDs)

---

*Wyoming classifies AIDS as a sexually transmitted disease. See Wyo. Stat. § 35-4-130
(Supp. 1989). It also requires reporting of HIV infection (telephone conversation
between Thomas Tierney and Roger Burr of the Wyoming Division of Health and
Medical Services AIDS Program, July 1990).

Appendix 13–B: Legal Assistance Resource List

This appendix lists organizations involved in AIDS-related legal work or that may be of particular use to legal advocates. The list is organized by issue and by region. In regions that do not have a legal-oriented organization, a community-based AIDS organization is listed. The list is based in part on the *Directory of Legal Resources for People With AIDS & HIV* (1991), published by the AIDS Coordination Project of the American Bar Association.

National Organizations

American Bar Association
AIDS Coordinating Committee
1800 M St. NW
Washington, DC 20036
(202) 331-2248

Canadian AIDS Society
1101-170 Laurier West
Ottawa, Canada K1P 5V5
(613) 230-3580

Center for Constitutional Rights
666 Broadway
New York, NY 10012
(212) 614-6464

Center for Women Policy Studies
2000 P St. NW, Suite 508
Washington, DC 20036
(202) 872-1770

Lambda Legal Defense & Education Fund
666 Broadway
New York, NY 10012
(212) 995-8585

Lambda Legal Defense & Education Fund
606 S. Olive St., Suite 580
Los Angeles, CA 90014
(213) 629-2728

National Association of People With AIDS
2025 I St. NW, Suite 1101
Washington, DC 20006
1-800-673-8538

National Center for Lesbian Rights
1663 Mission St., 4th Floor
San Francisco, CA 94103
(415) 621-0674

National Lawyers Guild AIDS Network
558 Capp Street
San Francisco, CA 94110
(415) 824-8884

National Minority AIDS Council
300 I St., 4th Floor
Washington, DC 20002
(202) 544-1076

American Civil Liberties Union

ACLU of Illinois
20 E. Jackson Blvd., Suite 1600
Chicago, IL 60604
(312) 427-7330

ACLU of the National Capitol Area
1400 20th St. NW
Washington, DC 20036
(202) 457-0800

ACLU National Office
AIDS and Civil Liberties Project
132 W. 43rd St.
New York, NY 10036
(212) 944-9800

ACLU chapters in all states may be contacted through the national office. The
following chapters have staff attorneys specializing in HIV-related issues.

ACLU of Northern California
1663 Mission St., Suite 460
San Francisco, CA 94103
(415) 621-2493

ACLU of Pennsylvania
P.O. Box 1161
Philadelphia, PA 19105
(215) 923-4357

ACLU of Southern California
1616 Beverly Blvd.
Los Angeles, CA 90026
(213) 977-9500

Child Law

National Center for Youth Law
114 Sansome St., Suite 900
San Francisco, CA 94104
(415) 543-3307

**National Legal Resource Center for Child Advocacy
and Protection**
1800 M St. NW
Washington, DC 20036
(202) 331-2250

Disability Rights

Disability Rights Education and Defense Fund
2212 6th St.
Berkeley, CA 94710
(510) 644-2555

National Association of Protection and Advocacy Systems
900 2nd St. NE, Suite 211
Washington, DC 20002
(202) 408-9514
(Also state centers with AIDS programs in California, Colorado, Florida,
Michigan, New York, Tennessee, and Texas)

Employment

Department of Fair Employment and Housing
State of California
30 Van Ness Ave., 3rd Floor
San Francisco, CA 94102
(415) 557-2005

Employment Law Center
1663 Mission St.
San Francisco, CA 94103
(415) 864-8848

Government

National AIDS Information Clearinghouse
1-800-458-5231
(CDC guidelines and other publications)

Office of Federal Contract Compliance Programs (OFCCP)
200 Constitution Ave. NW, Room C3325
Washington, DC 20210
(202) 523-9430
(Re: Federal contractor compliance with federal antidiscrimination law)

U.S. Department of Health and Human Services
Office for Civil Rights
330 Independence Ave. SW, Room 5400
Washington, DC 20201
(202) 619-0553
(Investigates cases of discrimination against people with handicaps, including HIV)

Health Law

American Public Health Association
1015 15th St. NW
Washington, DC 20005
(202) 789-5600

American Society of Law and Medicine
765 Commonwealth Ave., 16th Floor
Boston, MA 02215
(617) 262-4990

National Health Law Program
2639 S. La Cienega Blvd.
Los Angeles, CA 90034
(213) 204-6010
and
2025 M St. NW, Suite 400
Washington, DC 20036
(202) 887-5310

Housing

National Housing Law Project
1950 Addison Street
Berkeley, CA 94704
(510) 548-9400

Immigration

Center for Immigration Rights
48 St. Mark's Pl.
New York, NY 10009
(718) 899-4000

**Coalition for Immigration and Refugee Rights
and Services (CIRRS)**
HIV Task Force
995 Market St., Suite 1108
San Francisco, CA 94103
(415) 243-8215

Legalization Project
Volunteer Legal Services Program
Bar Association of San Francisco
685 Market St., Suite 700
San Francisco, CA 94105

National Immigration Project
National Lawyers Guild
14 Beacon St., Suite 506
Boston, MA 02108
(617) 227-9727

Traveler's Aid Society
74-09 37th Ave., Room 412
Jackson Heights, NY 10372
(718) 899-1233

Legislative

ACLU National Legislative Office
122 Maryland Ave. NE
Washington, DC 20002
(202) 544-1681

AIDS Action Council
2033 M St. NW, Suite 802
Washington, DC 20036
(202) 293-2886

Human Rights Campaign Fund
1012 14th St. NW, Suite 607
Washington, DC 20005
(202) 628-4160

National Gay and Lesbian Task Force
1517 U St. NW
Washington, DC 20009
(202) 332-6483

Military

Military Law Task Force
National Lawyers Guild
1168 Union St., Suite 202
San Diego, CA 92101
(619) 233-1701

Prisons

National Prison Project of the ACLU
1875 Connecticut Ave. NW, Suite 410
Washington, DC 20009
(202) 234-4830

Prisoners' Legal Services of New York
105 Chambers St., 5th Floor
New York, NY 10007
(212) 513-7373
(Offices in Albany, Plattsburgh, Poughkeepsie, Ithaca, and Buffalo)

14

Resources

National Resources

American Civil Liberties Union
AIDS and Civil Liberties Project
132 West 43rd Street
New York, NY 10036
(212) 944-9800

Will undertake AIDS civil rights litigation.

American Foundation for AIDS Research (AmFAR)
733 Third Avenue
New York, NY 10017-8901
(212) 682-7440

Publishes a clinical trials directory.

Center for Disease Control National AIDS Clearinghouse
1-800-458-5231 for information, resources, and referrals

1-800-243-7012 TDD (for hearing impaired)
(301) 217-0023 International
(301) 738-6616 fax
P.O. Box 6003
Rockville, MD 20849-6003

Database with more than 16,000 organizations that provide HIV and AIDS prevention, education, and social services. These include public health departments, community and social service organizations, hospitals, clinics, religious organizations, professional organizations and associations, and groups concerned about workplace issues.

Center for Disease Control National AIDS Hotline
1-800-342-AIDS or 1-800-342-2437 (English)
1-800-344-SIDA (Spanish)
1-800-AIDS-TTY (for hearing impaired)

Provides current and accurate information about HIV and AIDS to the general public—24-hour information as well as local hotline numbers where available.

Center for Substance Abuse Treatment
Rockwall II Building
5600 Fischers Lane
Rockville, MD 20857
(301) 443-5052
1-800-662-HELP (hotline for substance abuse treatment referrals)

Coalition of Hispanic and Health and
Human Services Organizations
1501 16th Street, NW
Washington, DC 20036
(202) 387-5000

This national organization's goal is to improve the health and well-being of all Hispanic communities in the United States by conducting national demonstration programs; coordinating research; and serving as a source of information, technical assistance, and policy analysis.

National Gay Rights Advocates
AIDS Civil Rights Project
540 Castro Street

San Francisco, CA 94114
Will assist with civil rights litigation.

National Institute of Allergy and Infectious Disease
Office of Communications
Building 31, Room 7-A-50
9000 Rockville Pike
Bethesda, MD 20892
(301) 496-5717

National Institute of Justice
AIDS Clearinghouse
1600 Reasearch Boulevard
Department F
Rockville, MD 20850
(301) 251-5500

National Institute of Mental Health
AIDS Program
5600 Fischers Lane, Room 1075
Rockville, MD 20857
(301) 443-6100

National Institutes of Health
Building 1, Room 126
9000 Rockville Pike
Bethesda, MD 20892
(301) 496-2433

Project Inform
1965 Market Street, Suite 220
San Francisco, CA 94103
1-800-822-7422
_____

National hotline for free information and distribution of materials for patients and providers.

Social Security Administration
U.S. Department of Health and Human Services
Hubert Humphrey Building, Room 716 G

200 Independence Avenue
Washington, DC 20201
1-800-772-1213

Specific information on Social Security Disability Insurance, Supplemental Security Income, Medicare; also will make appointments for local Social Security offices.

U.S. Conference of Mayors
AIDS Programs
1620 Eye Street, NW
Washington, DC 20006
(202) 293-7330

Publishes a national directory of AIDS service organizations.

State Resources

ALABAMA

Alabama AIDS Hotline: 1-800-228-0469

Alabama Department of Human Resources
Gordon Persons Administration Building
50 North Ripley Avenue
Montgomery, AL 36130-1801
(205) 242-1361

AIDS Task Force of Alabama
P.O. Box 55703
Birmingham, AL 35255
(205) 592-AIDS

Alabama Department of Public Health
HIV/AIDS Prevention and Control Division
Central Office
434 Monroe Street
Montgomery, AL 36130-3017
(205) 242-5838
(205) 242-5609

ALASKA

Alaska Hotline: 1-800-478-AIDS

Alaska AIDS Assistance Association
730 I Street, Suite 100
Anchorage, AK 99501
(907) 276-1400

Alaska Division of Public Assistance
400 Gambell Street
Anchorage, AK 99501
(907) 247-6524

State of Alaska AIDS/STD Program
Section of Epidemiology
Department of Health and Social Services
3601 C Street, Suite 576
Anchorage, AK 99524-0249
(907) 561-4406

ARIZONA

Arizona AIDS Information Line: (602) 234-2752

Arizona Spanish Speaking Community Information and Referral:
(602) 263-8856

Arizona AIDS Project
4460 North Central Avenue
Phoenix, AZ 85012-1850

Arizona Department of Health
3815 North Black Canyon Highway
Phoenix, AZ 85012
(602) 230-5819

Arizona Health Care Cost Containment System (Human Services)
3120 East Roosevelt Street
P.O. Box 5210
Phoenix, AZ 85010
(602) 495-3330

ARKANSAS

Arkansas AIDS Hotline: 1-800-364-2437/501-663-7833

Arkansas AIDS Foundation
5911 H Street
Little Rock, AR 72205

Arkansas Department of Health
Division of AIDS/STD
4815 West Markham Street
Little Rock, AR 72205
(501) 671-1462

CALIFORNIA

Hotline (Southern California): 1-800-922-2437/213-876-2437
Hotline (Northern California): 1-800-367-2437/415-863-2437

California Department of Health Services
Office of AIDS
830 S Street
P.O. Box 94234-7320
Sacramento, CA 95814
(916) 445-0553

COLORADO

Hotline: 1-800-333-2437/303-782-5276

Colorado AIDS Project
1576 Sherman Street
P.O. Box 18529
Denver, CO 80218
(303) 837-0166

Colorado Department of Health Services for AIDS/STD
4300 Cherry Creek Drive, South
Building A3
Denver, CO 80222-1530
(303) 692-2700

CONNECTICUT

Hotline: 203-566-1157

**Connecticut Department of Public Health
and Addiction Services**
AIDS Section
150 Washington Street
Hartford, CT 06106
(203) 566-5058

Connecticut Department of Social Services
Central Office
25 Sigourney Street
Hartford, CT 06106
1-800-842-1508/1-800-842-4524 TTD/TTY line (for hearing impaired)

DELAWARE

Hotline: 302-652-6776

Delaware Department of Health and Social Services
Division of Public Health
P.O. Box 637
Dover, DE 19903
(302) 739-3032

DISTRICT OF COLUMBIA

Hotline: 202-332-AIDS (Spanish)
(202) 328-9697 TTY (for hearing impaired)
(202) 797-3575

Agency for HIV/AIDS
1660 L Street, NW
Suite 700
Washington, DC 20036
(202) 673-6888
(202) 673-6703 TTY (for hearing impaired)

D.C. Income Maintenance Administration
645 H Street, NE
Washington, DC 20002
(202) 724-5190

GEORGIA

Hotline: 1-800-551-2728/404-876-9944

AIDS Atlanta
1132 West Peachtree, NE
Atlanta, GA 30309
(404) 872-0600

Department of Human Resources
Division of Public Health
868 Peachtree, NE
Atlanta, GA 30309
(404) 894-5307

HAWAII

Hotline: (Oahu) 1-800-321-1555
(neighboring islands) (808) 922-4787

Hawaii Department of Health
Communicable Disease Division
P.O. Box 3378
Honolulu, HI 96801
(808) 586-4580

IDAHO

Hotline: 1-800-833-2437

Idaho AIDS Foundation
P.O. Box 421
Boise, ID 83701
(208) 345-2277

Idaho Department of Health and Welfare
Idaho State AIDS/STD Program
450 West State Street
Boise, ID 83720

ILLINOIS

Hotline: 1-800-243-2437

Illinois Department of Public Health
AIDS Activities Section
160 North LaSalle, 7th Floor South
Chicago, IL 60601
(312) 814-4846 (Chicago)
(217) 524-5983 (Springfield)

INDIANA

Hotline: 1-800-848-AIDS

Indiana State Department of Health
Division of Acquired Diseases
1330 West Michigan Street
Indianapolis, IN 46206-1964
(317) 633-0893

IOWA

Hotline: 1-800-445-2437

Iowa Department of Public Health
Bureau of Infectious Diseases
Lucas State Office Building, Third Floor
Des Moines, IA 50319
(515) 242-5149

KANSAS

Kansas Department of Health and Environment
Bureau of Disease Control

Mills Building
109 S.W. 9th Street, Suite 605
Topeka, KS 66612-1271
(913) 296-6036
(913) 296-5587

KENTUCKY

Hotline: 1-800-654-2437

Kentucky Department for Health Services
Surveillance Section
275 East Main Street
Frankfort, KY 40621
(502) 564-3418
(502) 564-7243

Cabinet for Human Resources
275 East Main Street
Frankfort, KY 40621
(502) 564-4804

LOUISIANA

Hotline: 1-800-992-4379

Louisiana Department of Health and Human Resources
VD Control Section/AIDS Surveillance Sector
Box 60630
New Orleans, LA 70160
(504) 568-5275
(504) 568-5013

MAINE

Hotline: 1-800-851-2437

Maine Office on AIDS
157 Capitol Street
State House, Station II

Augusta, ME 04333
(207) 287-3707

MARYLAND

Hotline: 1-800-638-6252
Teen Hotline: 410-945-2437

Governor's Advisory Council on AIDS
201 West Preston Street, Third Floor
Baltimore, MD 21201
(410) 225-1663

Health Education Resource Organization
101 West Read Street, Suite 825
Baltimore, MD 21201
(410) 685-1180

Hotlines: (410) 945-2347
(410) 333-2437
1-800-638-6252
1-800-553-3140 TTD (for hearing impaired)

Maryland Department of Health
Maryland CARES
201 West Preston, Fourth Floor
Baltimore, MD 21201
(410) 333-2000

MASSACHUSETTS

Hotline: 1-800-235-2331/617-536-7733

AIDS Action Committee of Massachusetts
131 Clarendon Street
Boston, MA 02116
(617) 437-6200

Massachusetts Department of Public Health
AIDS Office

150 Tremont Street, 11th Floor
Boston, MA 02111
(617) 727-0368

MICHIGAN

Hotline: 1-800-872-2437

Michigan Department of Public Health
Special Office on AIDS Prevention
3423 North Logan/Martin Luther King Boulevard
P.O. Box 30195
Lansing, MI 48909
(517) 335-8371

MINNESOTA

Hotline: 1-800-248-2437

Minnesota AIDS Project
2025 Nicollett Avenue, S.E.
Suite 200
Minneapolis, MN 55404

Minnesota Department of Health
AIDS/STD Prevention Services
717 Delaware Street, S.E.
Minneapolis, MN 55440
(612) 623-5709 / (612) 623-5363 / (612) 623-5414

MISSISSIPPI

Hotline: 1-800-826-2961

Mississippi Department of Health
HIV/AIDS Prevention Program
2423 North State Street
P.O. Box 1700
Jackson, MS 39215-1700
(601) 960-7723

MISSOURI

Hotline: 1-800-533-2437

AIDS Foundation
214 South Central Street
Clayton, MO 63105
(314) 727-9181

Missouri Department of Health
Bureau of AIDS Prevention
1730 East Elm Street
P.O. Box 570
Jefferson City, MO 65101
(314) 751-6149 / (314) 751-6144 / (314) 751-6080

MONTANA

Hotline: 1-800-537-6187
Helpline: (406) 252-1212 (for referrals)

Montana Department of Health and Environmental Sciences
AIDS/STD Program
Cogswell Building
Helena, MT 59620
(406) 444-3565 / (404) 444-2457 / (404) 444-4748

NEBRASKA

Hotline: 1-800-782-2437

Nebraska AIDS Project
3642 Leavenworth Street
Omaha, NE 68105
(402) 342-4233

Nebraska Department of Health
301 Centennial Mall South
P.O. Box 95007
Lincoln, NE 68509
(402) 471-2937

NEVADA

Hotline: 1-800-842-AIDS

Nevada Department of Human Resources
Health Division
HIV/AIDS Program
505 East King Street—Room 304
Carson City, NV 89701
(702) 687-4800

NEW HAMPSHIRE

Hotline: 1-800-639-1122

New Hampshire AIDS Foundation
130 Middle Street
P.O. Box 59
Manchester, NH 03105-0059
(603) 623-0710

New Hampshire Health and Human Services
Office of Disease Prevention and Control
Health and Welfare Building
6 Hazen Drive
Concord, NH 03301-6527
(603) 271-4477 / (603) 241-4671

NEW JERSEY

Hotline: 1-800-624-2437

Hyacinth Foundation
103 Bayard Street
New Brunswick, NJ 08901
(908) 246-0204

Hotline: 1-800-443-0254

New Jersey Department of Health
AIDS Prevention and Control
363 West State Street

Trenton, NJ 08652-0363
(609) 984-6050 / (609) 984-6125

NEW MEXICO

Hotline: 1-800-545-2437

New Mexico AIDS Services, Inc.
1223 Saint Francis Drive, Suite C
Santa Fe, NM 87501-4033
(505) 984-0911

New Mexico Department of Epidemiology
New Mexico AIDS Task Force
1190 Saint Francis Drive, Room 1350
P.O. Box 26110
Santa Fe, NM 87502

NEW YORK

Hotline: 1-800-541-2437
New York City: (212) 447-8200

Gay Men's Health Crisis, Inc.
129 West 20th Street
New York, NY 10001
(212) 807-6664

Hotline: (212) 807-6655

New York City Human Resources Administration
Division of AIDS Services
11 West 13th Street, 5th Floor Intake
New York, NY 10001
(212) 645-7070 (AIDS Helpline)

New York State Department of Health
AIDS Institute
Corning Tower, Room 359
Albany, NY 12237
(518) 473-7542

5 Penn Plaza, Fourth Floor
New York, NY 10001
(212) 613-2492

NORTH CAROLINA

Hotline: 1-800-342-AIDS

North Carolina Department of Environment, Health,
and Natural Resources
HIV/STD Control Branch
P.O. Box 27687
Raleigh, NC 27611-7687
(919) 733-7301 / (919) 733-7081

NORTH DAKOTA

Hotline: 1-800-472-2180

North Dakota Department of Health
North Dakota AIDS Task Force
Division of Disease Control
Bismarck, ND 58505
(701) 224-2378 / (701) 224-3324

OHIO

Hotline: 1-800-342-2437

Ohio AIDS Task Force
Ohio Department of Health
Bureau of Preventative Medicine
246 High Street
Columbus, OH 43266-0588
(614) 466-5480

Ohio Department of Public Health
AIDS Activities Unit
P.O. Box 118
Columbus, OH 43266-0118
(614)466-0295 / (614)752-8201

OKLAHOMA

Hotline: 1-800-522-9054

Oklahoma State Health Department
AIDS Division
Division of Epidemiology
1000 N.E. Tenth Street
Oklahoma City, OK 73117-1299
(405) 271-4060 / (405) 271-4636

OREGON

Hotline: 1-800-777-2437

Cascade AIDS Project
620 S.W. 5th Avenue
Suite 300
Portland, OR 97204
(503) 223-5907 / (503) 233-7087 / (503) 223-0238

Oregon State Health Department
Office of Epidemiology
HIV Section
P.O. Box 231
Portland, OR 97207
(503) 731-4029

PENNSYLVANIA

Hotline: 1-800-662-6080
(215) 732-2437 (local calls)

Pennsylvania Department of Health
Bureau of HIV/AIDS
HNW Building, Room 913
P.O. Box 90
Harrisburg, PA 17108
(717) 783-0479

Pennsylvania Department of Public Welfare
Case Management Unit
P.O. Box 8021
Harrisburg, PA 17105-8021
1-800-692-7462
1-800-922-9384

RHODE ISLAND

Hotline: 1-800-726-3010

Rhode Island Department of Health
AIDS Program
3 Capitol Hill
Canon Building
75 Davis Street, Suite 106
Providence, RI 02908-5097
(401) 277-2320

Rhode Island Project AIDS (The Project)
95 Chestnut Street, 3rd Floor
Providence, RI 02903-4161
(401) 277-2320

SOUTH CAROLINA

Hotline: 1-800-322-2437

South Carolina Department of Health
    and Environmental Control
Bureau of Preventative Health Services
HIV/AIDS Division
Robert Mills Complex
P.O. Box 101106
Columbia, SC 29211
(803) 737-4110

SOUTH DAKOTA

Hotline: 1-800-592-1861

South Dakota Division of Public Health
Communicable Disease Program
523 East Capital Street
Pierre, SD 57501
(605) 773-3364

TENNESSEE

Hotline: 1-800-525-2437

Nashville Cares
700 Craighead Street, Suite 200
Nashville, TN 37204
(615) 385-1510

Tennessee Department of Health
AIDS Program
C2-221 Cordell Hull Building
Nashville, TN 34247-4947
(615) 741-7500

TEXAS

Hotline: 1-800-248-1091

Senate Committee on Health and Human Services
P.O. Box 12068
Sam Huston Building
Austin, TX 78711
(512) 463-0360

Texas Department of Health
Bureau of AIDS
1100 West 49th Street
Austin, TX 78756-3199
(512) 458-7304 / (512) 252-8012

UTAH

Hotline: 1-800-537-1046 (recording)

Utah AIDS Foundation
450 South 900 East
Room 205
P.O. Box 3373
Salt Lake City, UT 84102
(801) 487-2100

Utah Department of Health
Bureau of HIV/AIDS Prevention and Control
288 North 1460 West
P.O. Box 16660
Salt Lake City, UT 84116-0660
(801) 538-6096

VERMONT

Hotline: 1-800-882-2437

Vermont Cares
P.O. Box 5248
Burlington, VT 05402
(802) 863-2437 / 1-800-649-2437

Vermont Department of Health
Department of Epidemiology
AIDS Department
60 Main Street
P.O. Box 70
Burlington, VT 05402
(802) 863-7240 / (802) 863-7245

VIRGINIA

Hotline: 1-800-533-4148

Virginia Department of Health
Bureau of AIDS/STD

AIDS Activity Program
P.O. Box 2448, Room 112
Richmond, VA 23218

Virginia Department of Social Services
Richmond Regional Office
1604 Santa Rosa Road
Wythe Building, Suite 103
Richmond, VA 23229-5088
(804) 662-9743

WASHINGTON

Hotline: 1-800-272-2437

Washington State Department of Health
State Office on HIV/AIDS
Building 9
Olympia, WA 98504-7841
(206) 586-8329

Seattle AIDS Prevention Project
Seattle King County Department of Public Health
2124 4th Avenue, Fourth Floor
Seattle, WA 98121
(206) 296-4999

WEST VIRGINIA

Hotline: 1-800-642-8244

West Virginia Department of Health and Human Services
151 11th Avenue
South Charleston, WV 25303
(304) 348-2950

WISCONSIN

Hotline: 1-800-334-2437
Milwaukee: (414) 273-2437

Wisconsin Division of Health
HIV/AIDS Program
Section of Acute and Communicable Disease Epidemiology
1414 East Washington Avenue, Room 241
Madison, WI 53703
(608) 267-5287

WYOMING

Hotline: 1-800-327-3577

Wyoming AIDS Prevention Program
Hathaway Building, Room 475
2300 Capital Avenue
Cheyenne, WY 82002
(307) 777-5800
(717) 783-0479

Index

About the Authors

Laurie J. Andrews, RN, is the Study Coordinator for the AIDS Clinical Trials Unit at Yale University. She previously spent 10 years as the AIDS Coordinator at Hartford Hospital, where she worked with people with AIDS. She has received numerous awards for her leadership in the AIDS epidemic, including the Connecticut Department of Public Health and Addiction Services AIDS Leadership award, Greater Hartford Jaycees Civil Servant of the Year, and a joint award from the Connecticut Civil Liberties Union and the Connecticut State Gay and Lesbian Coalition for Civil Rights for her contributions to the community. She has served on the boards of AIDS Project/Hartford and Latinos/as Contra SIDA and is actively involved in professional organizations, such as the Association for Nurses in AIDS Care and the Connecticut Nurses Association HIV Task Force. In addition, she chairs the Health Services Committee of the Greater Hartford HIV Action Initiative. She received her bachelor's in nursing from Syracuse University and is completing a master's in public health from the University of Connecticut Health Center.

Larry B. Broisman, MD, is Director of the HIV/AIDS Clinic and Associate Attending, Section of General Internal Medicine at Hartford Hospital, Hartford, Connecticut. He is also an Assistant Clinical Professor in the Department of Medicine at the University of Connecticut and Director of Medical Ambu-

219

latory Education at Hartford Hospital. He received his medical degree from the University of Medicine and Dentistry of New Jersey at Newark. His internship and residency in general internal medicine were served at the Albert Einstein College of Medicine—Bronx Municipal Hospital Center, Bronx, New York. He is an active member of the Greater Hartford Ryan White Consortium Board and is involved with the Greater Hartford Action Initiative.

Laurie B. Novick, MHSA, BSW, has been involved in AIDS work since 1982. In 1983 she became the founding Executive Director of the AIDS Council of Northeastern New York, one of the first AIDS service organizations in the country outside of a major urban center. In 1985, she received the Distinguished Service Award from the Capital District Gay Community Council for her leadership in the epidemic. For 4 years she managed the client advocacy, financial assistance, and housing programs at the AIDS ACTION Committee of Massachusetts, Inc. She is presently the Coordinator of the Greater Hartford HIV Action Initiative, a regional coalition based in Hartford, Connecticut. She has also volunteered as a founding board member of the Community Research Initiative of New England and has served as a community advisory board member to the AIDS Clinical Trials Group in Boston. She received her master's degree in human service administration from Antioch, New England, and a bachelor's in social welfare from the State University of New York at Albany.

John D. Shanley, MD, received his doctor of medicine at UCLA, where he also did his residency in internal medicine and a fellowship in infectious disease. He was board certified in internal medicine in 1976 and in infectious diseases in 1978. He has been an Assistant Professor at the University of Iowa, the University of Connecticut Health Center, and the Veterans Administration Medical Center. He is presently Director of the Division of Infectious Diseases at the Newington VAMC, Professor of Medicine at the University of Connecticut Health Center, Director of the University of Connecticut Health Center Division of Infectious Diseases, and Director of the Infectious Diseases Fellowship Program at the University of Connecticut Health Center. In 1993, he was named to the Connecticut State Chair in Infectious Diseases. He is a member of a number of professional associations, including the Infectious Disease Society of America, the Connecticut Infectious Disease Society, the International Society for Viral Research, and the Association of Clinical Scientists. His research and publications have focused on infectious diseases, pathogenesis of viral diseases, the immunology and immunopathology of herpes viruses, and infections due to cytomegalovirus.

Printed in the United States
By Bookmasters